Cancer Chemotherapeutic Agents

Cancer Chemotherapeutic Agents

Handbook of Clinical Data

Mike R. Sather, R.Ph., M.S.
Chief, VA Cooperative Studies Program
Central Research Pharmacy
Veterans Administration Medical Center
Alburquerque, New Mexico

Charles E. Weber, Jr., Pharm.D.
Assistant Chief, Pharmacy Service
Veterans Administration Medical Center
Palo Alto, California
Adjunct Professor of Clinical Pharmacy
University of the Pacific
School of Pharmacy
Stockton, California

John Dennis Preston, Pharm.D.
Assistant Professor
Department of Pharmacy and Pharmaceutics
Medical College of Virginia
Richmond, Virginia

Gary H. Lyman, M.D.
Assistant Professor, Section
of Hematology/Oncology
Department of Internal Medicine
University of South Florida
College of Medicine
Tampa, Florida

Stephen M. Sleight, R.Ph.,M.S.
Chief, Pharmacy Service
Veterans Administration Medical Center
Lexington, Kentucky

Martinus Nijhoff Medical Division
The Hague — Boston — London
1979

Published by G.K. Hall & Co.
70 Lincoln Street
Boston, Massachusetts 02111

Sole distributor outside the USA, its dependencies, the Philippine Islands, and Canada:

Martinus Nijhoff Publishers
P.O.B. 566
2501 CN The Hague, The Netherlands

ISBN 90 247 2170 9

This publication is intended to serve merely as an outline guide for those skilled in chemotherapy. Care has been taken in compiling and checking the information; however, in NO circumstance should the information and protocols be used as a substitute for current medically accepted diagnostic and treatment procedures. The information is abbreviated and serves only to improve recall and assist in the normal diagnostic and therapeutic processes. Therapeutic decisions, including doses, intervals, and routes of administration, should be based on information contained in more comprehensive references. Neither the authors nor the publisher will be responsible for the continued currency of the information, for any inaccuracies, or any consequences of the clinical use of this material.

The authors wish to express their appreciation to Ms. Mary D. Allman and Miss Loretta A. Borah for their painstaking efforts in typing and proofreading the manuscript.

Contents

Cancer Chemotherapeutic Agents

Introduction

Cancer Chemotherapeutic Agents brings together from many diverse sources information relevant to the preparation and administration of drugs used in cancer chemotherapy. Drugs are listed alphabetically by nonproprietary name, and many of their trade names are identified. This is not, however, a comprehensive listing and should not be considered an endorsement of any product or manufacturer. This handbook has been prepared for use by physicians, pharmacists, and nurses involved in oncology. It should also prove to be particularly helpful to those health professionals who find themselves newly involved with cancer treatment in wards and clinics of health-care facilities. As cancer care rapidly expands throughout this country, more and more individuals find themselves at least peripherally involved. The authors sincerely hope this text will make that involvement easier.

1

Principles of Tumor Cell Biology

1. In preparation for division, all renewing cells go through a series of stages (the cell cycle) that includes G_1 (protein and RNA synthesis), S (DNA synthesis), G_2 (protein and RNA synthesis), and M (mitosis, cell division).
2. The *growth fraction* is the percentage of cells in a tumor that are in the cell cycle (proliferating pool).
3. Large differences in tumor doubling times in man cannot be explained on the basis of small differences in cell cycle times. Cells in the resting phase (G_0), tumor-cell death, and tumor-cell differentiation must be considered.
4. Normal cell growth is limited by certain genetic and epigenetic factors, such as various growth factors, nutritional needs, and cell-cell interactions.
5. Cells may lose all capacity to grow (static cells), resume growth on stimulation (expanding cells), or continuously replace effete elements (renewing cells).
6. The basic oncologic problem is the partial loss of control that would normally regulate expansion of a proliferating pool of cells.
7. Tumor size is directly proportional to the number of tumor cells, which is inversely proportional to the growth fraction.

8. A single unchallenged tumor cell can proliferate in an exponential fashion to kill the host. As the tumor size increases, cell proliferation slows, at a rate approximating a Gompertzian growth curve.
9. There is a normal host mechanism based on tumor-specific membrane antigens, which serves to initiate an immune response and eradicate small numbers of tumor cells.
10. Malignant disease becomes clinically manifest only when a large tumor burden is present (e.g., 10^8 cells or more).
11. Some, or perhaps most, tumors produce biochemical markers or fetal proteins, which may be detectable when other clinical evidence of tumor cells is absent.

Current incidence figures for carcinoma in the United States by site and sex are presented in Table 1.

References

Harriss, E. B., and Hoelzer, D. DNA synthesis time in leukemic cells as measured by the double labeling and percentage labeled mitosis methods. *Cell Tissue Kinet.* 4:433–41, 1971.

Lord, B.I. Measurement of the duration of DNA synthesis in erythroid cells of the bone marrow using a double labeling autoradiographic technique designed specifically for use with hemopoietic tissues. *Cell Tissue Kinet.* 3:13–19, 1970.

Tannock, I.F. A comparison of cell proliferation parameters in solid and ascites Ehrlich tumors. *Cancer Res.* 29:1527–34, 1969.

Young, R. C., and DeVita, V. T. Cell cycle characteristics of human solid tumors in-vivo. *Cell Tissue Kinet.* 3:285–90, 1970.

2

Principles of Cancer Chemotherapy

1. Chemotherapeutic agents act through first-order kinetics (fixed percentage of cell-kill), with subsequent survival inversely correlated with the initial tumor-cell mass.
2. All chemotherapeutic agents affect normal tissues as well as malignant cells. Renewing populations of cells, including bone marrow, gastrointestinal mucosa, and skin, are most severely affected.
3. Phases of chemotherapeutic management
   a. Supportive care only
   b. Palliation/symptom control
   c. Remission/induction
   d. Remission/consolidation
   e. Remission/maintenance
   f. Cure (adjuvant therapy)
4. Factors influencing chemotherapeutic responsiveness
   a. Type of malignancy
   b. Proliferative state of malignant cells
      (1) Growth fraction (percentage of cells in cycle)

(2) Rate of cell replication (doubling time)

c. Total burden of tumor cells

d. General condition of the host (nutrition)

5. Reasons for chemotherapeutic failure

a. Lack of active agents

b. Inappropriate doses, schedules, routes, and combinations, resulting in insufficient drug concentrations in malignant cells during a sensitive period of the cell cycle

c. Development of tumor-cell resistance

(1) Decreased cell uptake

(2) Altered target enzyme

(3) Decreased drug activation

(4) Increased drug deactivation

(5) Increased DNA repair

(6) Increased use of salvage pathways

d. Increased cell replication (new steady state)

e. Poor distribution to malignant cells because of prior radiation therapy or surgery

f. Severe toxicity

g. Immunosuppression/teratogenesis/carcinogenesis

h. Poor functional/nutritional status

i. Advanced age

6. Recent advances in cancer chemotherapy

a. Introduction of new active drugs

b. Improved understanding of tumor-cell and normal-cell kinetics

c. Improved ability to control drug toxicity

d. Improved supportive care
   (1) Antibiotics
   (2) Blood component therapy
   (3) Dialysis
   (4) Total parenteral nutrition
e. Use of regional chemotherapy (e.g., intracavitary instillation, intra-arterial or intrathecal administration)
f. Use of chemotherapy early in the course of the disease (e.g., adjuvant chemotherapy)
g. Use of combination chemotherapy
   (1) Empiric (trial and error)
   (2) Rational
      (a) Different mechanisms of action: depletion of end-product by sequential, concurrent, or complementary inhibition
      (b) Different cell-cycle actions: nonspecific (alkylators), cycle-specific (antibiotics), and phase-specific (M–vinca alkaloids; S–antimetabolites)
      (c) Different toxicities: drugs with minimal bone marrow toxicity (e.g., vincristine, bleomycin, *cis*-platinum, L-asparaginase, and hormones)
      (d) Different temporal onset of toxicity: early onset (hydroxyurea and antimetabolites) and late onset (nitrosoureas and other alkylators)
h. Use of multimodality therapy for greatest tumor reduction (surgery, radiation therapy, endocrine therapy, chemotherapy, and immunotherapy)
i. Multidisciplinary management (includes pathologists, surgical oncologists, radiation oncologists, medical oncologists, and clinical pharmacists)

j. Use of biologic markers and fetal antigens to follow subclinical disease

k. Improved tumor classification (pathologic and staging)

Tumor, Node, and Metastases (TNM)

Tumor:	T_0	=	no evidence of tumor
	T_{is}	=	*in situ*
	T_{1-4}	=	increasing tumor size or local extension
Node:	N_0	=	no nodal disease
	N_{1-2A}	=	palpable regional lymph nodes (no metastases suspected)
	$N_{1-2B,3}$	=	palpable regional lymph nodes (metastases suspected)
Metastases:	M_0	=	no metastases
	M_1	=	metastases present

l. Use of drugs in pulse regimens (intermittent)

(1) Possible recruitment of tumor cells

(2) Recovery of normal cells more rapid than that of malignant cells

m. Use of maintenance chemotherapy

n. Use of controlled, prospective randomized clinical trials

o. Promising but unproven methods

(1) Cell synchronization

(2) Chemoimmunotherapy

(3) Biochemical predictive tests (cell-culture screening methods)

(4) Preoperative chemotherapy

7. Responsive malignant disorders

   a. Curable (normal life expectancy) with chemotherapy alone in some patients

      (1) Wilms' tumor

      (2) Ewing's sarcoma

      (3) Embryonal rhabdomyosarcoma

      (4) Acute lymphocytic leukemia (childhood) (ALL)

      (5) Burkitt's lymphoma

      (6) Choriocarcinoma

      (7) Hodgkin's disease

      (8) Testicular cancer

      (9) Histiocytic lymphoma

      (10) Skin cancer

   b. Curable in adjuvant setting (for residual microscopic disease)

      (1) Neuroblastoma

      (2) Breast cancer (probable)

      (3) Small-cell carcinoma of the lung (probable)

      (4) Osteogenic sarcoma

      (5) Retinoblastoma

   c. Palliation with significant percentage of objective responders

      (1) Head and neck cancer

      (2) Acute myelogenous leukemia (AML)

      (3) Lymphocytic lymphoma

      (4) Multiple myeloma

      (5) Carcinoma of the bladder

(6) Soft-tissue sarcomas

(7) Insulinoma

(8) Adenocarcinoma of the ovary

(9) Chronic lymphocytic leukemia (CLL)

(10) Chronic myelogenous leukemia (CML)

(11) Endometrial carcinoma

(12) Carcinoid

Chemotherapy remains useful in disease palliation for symptom control (e.g., pain relief and psychological support). Note that administration of live-virus vaccines should be avoided unless clearly indicated. Other vaccinations, if indicated, should be administered in the intervals between courses of chemotherapy.

References

Carter, S. K., and Soper, W. T. Integration of chemotherapy into combined modality treatment of solid tumors: I. The overall strategy. *Cancer Treat. Rev.* 1:1–13, 1974.

DeVita, V. T., and Schein, P. S. The use of drugs in combination for the treatment of cancer. Rationale and results. *N. Engl. J. Med.* 288:988–1006, 1973.

DeVita, T. T.; Young, R. C.; and Cantellos, G. D. Combination versus single agent chemotherapy: A review of the basis for selection of drug therapy of cancer. *Cancer* 35:98–110, 1975.

Henderson, E. S., and Samach, R. J. Evidence that drugs in multiple combinations have materially advanced the treatment of human malignancies. *Cancer Res.* 29:2272–80, 1969.

Klein, H. O., and Lennartz, K. J. Chemotherapy after synchronization of tumor cells. *Semin. Hematol.* 11:203–27, 1974.

Livingston, R. B., and Carter, S. K. *Single agents in cancer chemotherapy.* New York: Plenum Press, 1970.

Martin, E. S.; Fugman, R. A.; and Hayworth, P. Surgery, cancer chemotherapy, host defenses and tumor size. *J. Natl. Cancer Inst.* 29:817–34, 1962.

Perloff, M., and Holland, J. D. Surgical adjuvant chemotherapy. *Annu. Rev. Med.* 28:475–88, 1977.

Sartorelli, A. C. Some approaches to the therapeutic exploitation of metabolic sites of vulnerability of neoplastic cells. *Cancer Res.* 29:2292–99, 1969.

Schabel, F. M., Jr. Concepts of systemic treatment of micrometastases. *Cancer* 35:15–24, 1975.

Silver, R. T.; Young, R. C.; and Holland, J. F. Some new aspects of modern cancer chemotherapy. *Am. J. Med.* 63:772–87, 1977.

Skipper, H. E.; Shabel, F. M.; and Wilcox, W. S. Experimental evaluation of potential anticancer agents XIII. On the criteria and kinetics associated with "curability" of experimental leukemia. *Cancer Chemother. Rep.* 35:1–111, 1964.

3

Principles of Cancer Chemotherapy Trials

1. Preclinical studies
   a. Animal models — efficacy, pharmacology, and toxicity of new drugs should be determined in a number of animal species
   b. L1210 leukemia (specialized rat animal model used for testing new drug activity)
   c. P 388 leukemia (specialized rat animal model used for testing new drug activity)
2. Clinical trials
   a. Phase 1 — pharmacology and dose toleration (maximum tolerated dose)
   b. Phase 2 — survey signal tumors for antitumor activity (objective response)
   c. Phase 3 — comparative clinical trial (objective response, survival)
   d. Phase 4 — adjuvant trial (survival)
3. Parameters to follow
   a. Response rate

(1) Complete remission — disappearance of all evidence of disease

(2) Partial objective response — greater than 50% reduction in the sum of the products of the two longest perpendicular diameters of all measurable disease

(3) Stable disease — less than 50% reduction in the sum of the products of the two longest perpendicular diameters of all measurable disease and less than a 25% increase in the product of the two perpendicular diameters of any measurable lesion

(4) Progressive disease — greater than 25% increase in the product of the two longest perpendicular diameters of any measurable lesion

b. Duration of response — time from first noted response to evident progressive disease

c. Survival

(1) Median survival — real or projected time required for 50% of patients to die

(2) Timed survival — percentage of patients surviving for a definite period of time (e.g., 1 year)

(3) Quality of survival

(a) Performance/activities

(b) Pain control

(c) Treatment toxicity

(d) Alertness

(e) Social support

(f) Meaningfulness

(g) Deformity

(h) Duration of hospitalization

4. Elements of clinical protocols
   a. Background and rationale (review of previous experience)
   b. Objectives of study
   c. Eligibility requirements (patient selection)
   d. Study design (including schematics)
   e. Stratification by independent prognostic factors
   f. Treatment to be administered
   g. Treatment modification
   h. Treatment preparation, formulation, and storage
   i. Data to be collected
   j. Criteria of response
   k. Statistical considerations
      (1) Duration of study
      (2) Patient numbers
   l. Informed consent
   m. Record forms
   n. Principal investigator
5. Difficulties
   a. Interpreting results of clinical trials
      (1) Bias (use randomization)
      (2) Historical controls (use concurrent controls)
      (3) Comparability of groups (use stratification)
   b. Evaluation of patients and protocol compliance (include all patients)
      (1) Multiple institutions (limit institutions and investigators)

(2) Small numbers of patients (limit number of randomization and stratification groups)

(3) Statistical fallacies

References

Byar, D. P.; Simon R. M.; Friedewald, R. T.; Schlesselman, J. J.; DeMets, D. L.; Ellenberg, J. H.; Gail, M. H.; and Ware, J. H. Randomized clinical trials: perspectives on some recent ideas. *N. Engl. J. Med.* 295:74–80, 1976.

Carter, S. K., and Soper, W. T. Integration of chemotherapy into combined modality treatment of solid tumors. I. The overall strategy. *Cancer Treat. Rev.* 1:1–13, 1974.

Feinstein, A. R.; Pritchett, J. A.; and Schimpff, C. R. The epidemiology of cancer therapy. II. The clinical course: data decision and temporal demarcations. *Arch. Intern. Med.* 123:323–44, 1969.

Gehan, E. A., and Schneiderman, M. A. Experimental design of clinical trials. In *Cancer Medicine,* ed. J. F. Holland, and E. Frei, III. Philadelphia: Lea and Febiger, 1973.

Golden, A.; Serpick, A. A.; and Mantel, N. Experimental screening procedures and clinical predictability. *Cancer Chemother. Rep.* 50:173, 1966.

Homan, E. R. Quantitative relationships between toxic dose of antitumor chemotherapeutic agents in animals and man. *Cancer Chemother. Rep.* 3:13–19, 1972.

Owens, A. H. Predicting anti-cancer drug effects in man from animal laboratory studies. *J. Chronic Dis.* 15:223–28, 1962.

Peto, R.; Pike, M. C.; Armtage, P.; Breslow, N. E.; Cox, D. R.; Howard, S. V.; Mantel, N.; McPherson, K.; Peto, J.; and Smith, P. G. Design and analysis of randomized clinical trials requiring prolonged observation of each patient. I. Introduction and design. *Brit. J. Cancer* 34:585–612, 1976.

Rudnick, S., and Capizzi, R. L. The conduct of therapeutic trials in cancer medicine. *Semin. Oncol.* 4:255–58, 1977.

Schneiderman, M. A. How do you know you've done any better? *Cancer* 35:64–69, 1975.

4

Classification of Agents

1. Alkylating Agents
   a. Nitrogen Mustards
      (1) Chlorambucil (Leukeran®)
      (2) Cyclophosphamide (Cytoxan®)
      (3) Mechlorethamine (Mustargen®)
      (4) Melphalan (Alkeran®)
      *(5) Uracil Mustard
   b. Ethylenimines
      *(1) Triethylenemelamine (TEM)
      *(2) Triethylenethiophosphoramide (Thiotepa®)
   c. Alkyl Sulfonates
      (1) Busulfan (Myleran®)
   d. Nitrosoureas
      (1) Carmustine (BCNU, BiCNU®)
      (2) Lomustine (CCNU, CeeNU®)
      (3) Semustine (Methyl-CCNU®)
      (4) Streptozotocin

e. Triazenes

(1) Dacarbazine (DTIC®)

f. Miscellaneous

(1) *Cis*-diamminedichloroplatinum (Platinol®)

2. Antimetabolites

a. Folic Acid Analogues

(1) Methotrexate (Methotrexate®)

b. Pyrimidine Analogues

*(1) Azaribine (Triazure)

(2) Cytarabine (Cytosar®)

(3) 5-Fluorouracil (Fluorouracil®)

c. Purine Analogues

(1) 6-Mercaptopurine (Purinethol®)

(2) 6-Thioguanine

d. Miscellaneous

(1) 5-Azacytidine

3. Natural Products

a. Vinca Alkaloids

(1) Vinblastine (Velban®)

(2) Vincristine (Oncovin®)

b. Antibiotics

(1) Bleomycin (Blenoxane®)

(2) Dactinomycin (Cosmegen®)

(3) Daunorubicin (Cerutidine®)

(4) Doxorubicin (Adriamycin®)

(5) Mithramycin (Mithracin®)

(6) Mitomycin C (Mutamycin®)

c. Enzymes

(1) L-Asparaginase (ELSpar®)

4. Hormones

a. Adrenocorticosteroids

(1) Prednisone

b. Progestins

*(1) Hydroxyprogesterone Caproate (Delalutin®)

(2) Medroxyprogesterone Acetate (Provera®)

(3) Megestrol Acetate (Megace®)

*(4) Norethisterone Acetate

c. Estrogens

(1) Chlorotrianisene (Tace®)

(2) Diethylstilbestrol (Diethylstilbestrol®, DES®)

*(3) Ethinyl Estradiol (Estinyl®)

d. Antiestrogens

(1) Tamoxifen Citrate (Nolvadex®)

*(2) Nafoxidine

e. Androgens

*(1) Calusterone

*(2) Drostanolone Proprionate

(3) Fluoxymesterone (Halotestin®)

*(4) Testolactone (Teslac®)

(5) Testosterone Cypionate

(6) Testosterone Enanthate

(7) Testosterone Proprionate (Oreton®)

5. Miscellaneous Agents
    a. Substituted Urea
        (1) Hydroxyurea (Hydrea®)
    b. Methylhydrazine Derivative
        (1) Procarbazine (Matulane®)
    c. Adrenocortical Suppressant
        *(1) Mitotane (Lysodren®)
    d. Hexamethylmelamine

*Not referred to in text.

Note: Classification adapted from P. Calabresi and R. E. Parks, Jr., Chemotherapy of Neoplastic Diseases, in *The Pharmacological Basis of Therapeutics,* 5th ed., ed. L. S. Goodman and A. Gilman (New York: Macmillan Publishing Company, 1975), pp. 1250–52; S. E. Salmon, Malignant Disorders, in *Current Medical Diagnosis and Treatment,* 17th ed., ed. M. A. Krupp and M. J. Chatton (Los Altos, Cal.: Lange Medical Publications, 1978), pp. 1008–9; and A. Clarysse and G. Mathe, Malignant Diseases, in *Drug Treatment: Principles and Practice of Clinical Pharmacology and Therapeutics,* ed. G. S. Avery (Acton, Mass.: Publishing Sciences Group, 1976), pp. 717–70.

5

Drug Monographs

L-ASPARAGINASE

Trade Name
Elspar®

Classification Category
Natural Product (Enzyme)

Dosage Forms & Route of Administration
10,000 units/vial; IV push, IV infusion, or IM

Mechanism of Action
Hydrolyzes L-asparagine, which sensitive tumor cells are incapable of synthesizing. Exploits a metabolic difference between neoplastic and normal tissues.

Indications, Dosage & Duration of Treatment
Acute lymphoblastic leukemia: 1,000 IU/kg every day for 10–14 days IV, or 6,000 IU/M² 3 times weekly for 3–4 weeks IM.

Rate of Administration

Absorption, Metabolism, Excretion

Onset, Duration of Action, $T_{1/2}$

Side Effects, Toxicity

Anaphylaxis (10%), hypersensitivity reactions (25%), pancreatitis (7%), CNS toxicity (30%), renal toxicity (34%), hepatotoxicity (50-100%; severe less than 5%), decrease in fibrinogen and other clotting factors (60–100%; clinical bleeding less than 1%), fever (25%), weight loss (25%), and nausea and vomiting (30%).

All toxicities are significantly worse in adult patients than in children.

Contraindications

Hypersensitivity to the drug.

Clinically Significant Drug Interactions

Notes

Because of the very high incidence of sensitization, the enzyme should not be given for a second induction, extended periods, or intermittently. Epinephrine (0.5 ml), hydrocortisone (100 mg), and oxygen by mask should be available.

The drug should be used only in acute lymphoblastic leukemia.

A rise in BUN and ammonia is due to action of the enzyme and is not evidence of toxicity.

The drug has essentially no bone marrow toxicity.

Store in refrigerator. Mix with 5 ml Sterile Water for Injection, U.S.P., or Sodium Chloride for Injection, U.S.P. Discard 6 hours after mixing. Use clear solution only.

References

Adamson, R. N., and Fabro, S. Antitumor activity and other biological properties of L-asparaginase: a review. *Cancer Chemother. Rev.* 52:617–26, 1968.

Broome, J. D. Studies of the mechanism of tumor inhibition of L-asparaginase. *J. Exp. Med.* 127:1055–72, 1968.

Burchenal, J. H., and Karnofsky, D. A. Clinical evaluation of L-asparaginase: introduction. *Cancer* 25:241–42, 1970.

Capizzi, R. L.; Bertino, J. R.; and Handschumacher, R. E. L-Asparaginase. *Annu. Rev. Med.* 21:433–44, 1970.

Capizzi, R. L.; Bertino, J. R.; Skeel, R. T.; Creasey, W. A.; Zares, R.; Olayon, C.; Peterson, R. G.; and Handschumacher, R. E. L-Asparaginase: clinical, biochemical, pharmacological, and immunological studies. *Ann. Intern. Med.* 74:893–901, 1971.

Cooney, D. A., and Handschumacher, R. E. L-Asparaginase and L-asparagine metabolism. *Annu. Rev. Pharmacol.* 10:421–40, 1970.

National Cancer Institute, *L-Asparaginase (NSC-109229).* Drug Monograph, Bethesda, Maryland, 1976.

Newton, W. A.; Ertel, J. J.; Nesbit, M. E.; Thatcher, G. L.; Karon M.; and Hammond, D. Effective dose of L-asparaginase in acute leukemia. *Proc. Am. Assoc. Res.* 14:78, 1973.

Oettgen, H. F.; Old, L. J.; Boyse, E. A.; Campbell, H. A.; Philips, F. S.; Clarkson, B. D.; Tallal, L.; Leeper, R. D.; Schwartz, M. K.; and Kim, J. H. Inhibition of leukemias in man by L-asparaginase. *Cancer Res.* 27:2619–13, 1967.

Whitecar, J. P., Jr.; Bodey, G. P.; Harris, J. E.; and Freirich, E. J. L-Asparaginase. *N. Engl. J. Med.* 282:732–34, 1970.

5-AZACYTIDINE

Trade Name
(Investigational NSC-102816)

Classification Category
Antimetabolite (Miscellaneous)

Dosage Forms & Route of Administration
100-mg vials; IV push, IV infusion

Mechanism of Action
Four mechanisms have been proposed:

a. Incorporation of 5-azacytidine into DNA following phosphorylation.

b. Incorporation of 5-azacytidine into RNA and hence interference with protein synthesis.

c. Competition for uridine kinase.

d. Inhibition of orotidylic acid decarboxylase.

Indications, Dosage & Duration of Treatment
To induce remission in acute granulocytic leukemia, use 150–200 mg/M^2/day for 5 days as a single rapid injection, or administer 150–200 mg/M^2/day as a continuous infusion for 5 days, changing the infusion solutions every 3 to 4 hours to avoid loss of drug potency secondary to drug decomposition.

Rate of Administration
Rapid IV injection or continuous 24-hour infusion.

Absorption, Metabolism, Excretion
Requires uridine-cytidine kinase for activation.
Ninety percent of the drug is excreted in the urine within 24 hours.

Onset, Duration of Action, $T_{1/2}$
$T_{1/2}$ after IV injection is 3.5 hours.

Side Effects, Toxicity
Nausea, vomiting, diarrhea, leukopenia, thrombocytopenia, anemia, abnormal liver-function tests, hepatic coma (rare), fever, rash, stomatitis, hypotension, and neuromuscular damage.

Contraindications
Should not be started in patients with preexisting drug-induced bone marrow suppression. Contraindicated in patients with hepatic metastases or serum albumin of less than 3 grams percent.

Clinically Significant Drug Interactions

Notes
Do not reconstitute with 5% Dextrose Injection. U.S.P. Lactated Ringer's is preferred.

References

Karon, M.; Sieger, L.; Leinbrook, S.; Finklestein, J. Z.; Nesbit, M. E.; and Swaney, J. J. 5-azacytidine: a new agent active for the treatment of acute leukemia. *Blood* 42:359-65, 1973.

National Cancer Institute. *5-azacytidine (NSC-102816).* Drug Monograph. Bethesda, Maryland, 1976.

BLEOMYCIN

Trade Name
Blenoxane®

Classification Category
Natural Product (Antibiotic)

Dosage Forms & Route of Administration
15 units/ampul; IV, IM, or SC

Mechanism of Action
Alters DNA and inhibits DNA synthesis, with some evidence of lesser inhibition of RNA and protein synthesis. Blocks cells at the G_2/M interface.

Indications, Dosage & Duration of Treatment
Lymphomas, testicular tumors, and squamous-cell carcinomas of skin, penis, vulva, head, and neck: 10–20 units/M^2 IV or IM 1 or 2 times/week; because of the possibility of anaphylactoid reaction (1% incidence), start with 2 units or less for first 2 doses in lymphoma.

Rate of Administration
Slow IV push for over a period of 10 minutes. IV infusion over 15–30 minutes, or slow infusion over 24 hours.

Absorption, Metabolism, Excretion
Largely excreted by the kidneys (20-40% as active drug).
Degraded intracellularly by an aminopetidase not found in skin and lungs.

Onset, Duration of Action, $T_{½}$
$T_{½}$ = 15–60 minutes; $T_{½}$ is prolonged in patients with impaired renal function.

Side Effects, Toxicity
Fever (4-6 hours) and chills (30%), anorexia, vomiting (15%), anaphylaxis, local pain or phlebitis (infrequent), skin hyperpigmentation or thickening (finger tips, soles, and palms) (10%), ulceration, rash, peeling, alopecia (60%), nail change, and pneumonitis (10%) with dyspnea, rales, and infiltrate (can progress to fibrosis) (1%). Pulmonary complications are more common in patients over 50, in patients who

are given more than 250 units/M^2 total dose or 25 units/M^2 single dose, and in those with prior lung disease or radiotherapy. They are unpredictable and may occur at a lower dose when bleomycin is used in combination with other antineoplastic agents. Discontinue the drug if there is a significant loss of pulmonary function.

Contraindications
Hypersensitivity to the drug, significant pulmonary disease.

Clinically Significant Drug Interactions

Notes
Watch for hypersensitivity in lymphoma with the first or second dose. Use extreme caution in presence of renal or pulmonary disease. Start in the hospital under observation. Do not exceed a total dose of 400 units.

The drug is virtually free of bone marrow toxicity, but it can cause skin changes as well as dose-related pulmonary toxicity that may progress to fibrosis. The drug accumulates in skin and lung tissue.

Store at room temperature. Reconstitution: IM or SC — 3–5 ml of Sterile Water for Injection, U.S.P., Sodium Chloride for Injection, U.S.P., or 5% Dextrose Injection, U.S.P.; IV infusion — 50–100 ml 5% Dextrose Injection, U.S.P., or Sodium Chloride for Injection, U.S.P. (infuse over 15–30 min); IV push — dissolve with 5 ml Sodium Chloride for Injection, U.S.P., or 5% Dextrose Injection, U.S.P., for a concentration of 3 units/ml to be administered over 10 minutes. The solution is stable for 24 hours at room temperature after reconstitution.

Observe for possible hypotension, fever, or anaphylaxis after administration.

Liver and kidney functions should be monitored.

References

Clinical Screening Group of EORTC. Study of the clinical efficiency of bleomycin in human cancer. *Brit. Med. J.* 2:643–45, 1970.

Holoye, P.Y.; Leura, M. A.; Macky, B.; and Bedrossian, C. W. M. Bleomycin hypersensitivity pneumonitis. *Ann. Intern. Med.* 88:47–49, 1978.

Shastri, S.; Slaton, R. E.; Walter, J.; Perlia, C. P.; and Taylor, S. G. Clinical study with bleomycin. *Cancer* 28:1142–46, 1971.

Yagoda, A.; Mukherji, B.; Young, C.; Etcubanas, E.; Lamonte, C.; Smith, J. R.; Tan, C. T. C.; and Krakoff, I. H. Bleomycin, an antitumor antibiotic. Clinical experience in 274 patients. *Ann. Intern. Med.* 77:861–70, 1972.

BUSULFAN

Trade Name
Myleran®

Classification Category
Alkylating Agent (Alkyl Sulfonate)

Dosage Forms & Route of Administration
2-mg oral tablets

Mechanism of Action
Alkylating agent (cross-linking of DNA)

Indications, Dosage & Duration of Treatment
Chronic granulocytic leukemia: daily dose of 4–8 mg until leukocyte count falls to 50% of original level, then reduce dosage (maintenance dose is 1–3 mg daily).

Rate of Administration

Absorption, Metabolism, Excretion
The drug is absorbed well (blood levels obtained within 0.5–2 hours), metabolized in minutes to methanesulfonic acid, and excreted by the kidneys (10–50% in 24 hours).

Onset, Duration of Action, $T_{1/2}$

Side Effects, Toxicity
Nausea, vomiting, diarrhea, alopecia, hyperuricemia, amenorrhea, sterility, impotence, glossitis, cheilosis, bone marrow depression, pulmonary fibrosis, cataracts, wasting syndrome (weight loss, hypotension, and pigmentation), and gynecomastia.

Contraindications
Prolonged bone marrow suppression.

Clinically Significant Drug Interactions

Notes

References

Hyman, G. A., and Gellhorn, A. Myleran therapy in malignant neoplastic disease. *J. A. M. A.* 161:844–49, 1956.

Vadopick, H. A.; Hamilton, H. E.; Jackson, H. B.; Peng, C. T.; and Sheets, R. F. Studies on the fate of tritiated busulfan *J. Clin. Invest.* 42:989, 1963.

CARMUSTINE (BCNU)

Trade Name
BiCNU®

Classification Category
Alkylating Agent (Nitrosourea)

Dosage Forms & Route of Administration
100-mg vial; IV infusion

Mechanism of Action

a. Alkylation by formation of diazohydroxide and/or 2-chlorethylamine.

b. Selective interference with the utilization of histidine in 1-carbon metabolism in *de novo* purine synthesis through inhibition of formimino-transferase or cyclodeaminase.

c. Increased NADase activity and decrease in concentration of NAD^+ in tumor cells.

d. Decreased DNA nucleotidyl-transferase activity.

Indications, Dosage & Duration of Treatment
Hodgkin's disease: when used as a single agent, 100 mg/M^2 to be repeated every 6 weeks, or daily injections of 100 mg/M^2 on successive days. If agent is to be used in combination, 75–100 mg/M^2 for one dose to be repeated every 6 weeks. Possibly effective in glioblastoma multiforme, multiple myeloma, and gastrointestinal malignancies.

Rate of Administration
Slow infusion rate to prevent local pain (over 1–2 hours in 100–150 ml 5% Dextrose Injection, U.S.P.).

Absorption, Metabolism, Excretion
Rapidly degraded by microsomal enzymes in the liver and slowly excreted in the urine (30% in 24 hours and 60–70% within 96 hours). Some enterohepatic circulation probably occurs.

Onset, Duration of Action, $T_{1/2}$
The drug is cleared from the plasma in 15 minutes after IV administration. Significant CSF concentration occurs almost immediately.

Side Effects, Toxicity

Nausea and vomiting 4–6 hours after administration; burning pain along vein; facial flushing; cumulative myelosuppression, including thrombocytopenia (4–5 weeks) and leukopenia (5–6 weeks); occasional renal toxicity (transient), hepatic toxicity (mild and reversible), and optic neuritis.

Contraindications

Consider alternate therapy or reduced dosage in patients with impaired bone marrow function. Contraindicated in patients with previous hypersensitivity.

Clinically Significant Drug Interactions

Notes

Over 50% objective response in patients with Hodgkin's disease has been reported, often after alkylating agents and vinca alkaloids have failed. A lesser degree of activity has been noted in the other lymphomas and in some solid tumors.

The drug is highly lipid-soluble and penetrates the blood-brain barrier (limited success with brain tumors).

Consider the use of antiemetics.

Store in refrigerator. Dissolve with 3 ml absolute alcohol and then 27 ml Sterile Water for Injection, U. S. P. The resulting solution contains 3.3 mg/ml of BCNU in 10% ethanol with a pH of 5.6–6.0 and can be further diluted with Sodium Chloride for Injection, U.S.P., or 5% Dextrose Injection, U.S.P. Discard 2 hours after mixing. Avoid contact with skin (causes brown spots). Alcohol diluent may cause flushing and local discomfort.

References

Carter, S. K., and Newman, J. W. Nitrosoureas: 1,3-*bis*-(-2-chloroethyl)-1-nitrosourea (NSC-409962; BCNU) and 1-(2-chloroethyl)-3-cyclohexyl-1-nitrosourea (NSC-79037; CCNU). Clinical brochure. *Cancer Chemother. Rep.* 1:115–51, 1968.

Lessner, H. E. BCNU (1,3-*bis*-(2-chloroethyl)-1-nitrosourea). Effects on advanced Hodgkin's disease and other neoplasia. *Cancer* 22:451–56, 1968.

Wasserman, T. H.; Slavik, M.; and Carter, S. K. Clinical comparison of nitrosoureas. *Cancer* 36:1258–68, 1975.

Wheeler, G. P., and Chumley, S. Alkylating activity of 1,3-*bis*-(2-chloroethyl) - 1-nitrosourea and related compounds. *J. Med. Chem.* 10:259–61, 1967.

Wilson, C. B.; Boldery, E. B.; and Enot, K. J. 1,3-*bis*-(2-chloroethyl)-1-nitrosourea (NSC-409962) in the treatment of brain tumors. *Cancer Chemother. Rep.* 54:273–81, 1970.

Young, R. C.; DeVita, V. T.; Serpick, A. A.; and Canellos, G. P. Treatment of advanced Hodgkin's disease with [1,3-*bis*-(2-chloroethyl)-1-nitrosourea] BCNU. *N. Engl. J. Med.* 285:475–79, 1971.

CHLORAMBUCIL

Trade Name
Leukeran®

Classification Category
Alkylating Agent (Nitrogen Mustard)

Dosage Forms & Route of Adminstration
2-mg oral tablets

Mechanism of Action
Alkylating Agent (cross-linking of DNA)(see mechlorethamine monograph).

Indications, Dosage & Duration of Treatment
The greatest clinical usefulness is in chronic lymphocytic leukemia: 0.1–0.2 mg/kg (maximum 14 mg) in a single daily dose before breakfast for 3–6 weeks; follow with blood count weekly, and adjust dosage as the white blood count diminishes (e.g., below 25,000/cu mm). When the white blood count falls to normal or near normal, stop the drug or reduce it to maintenance dose (2 mg daily or 6–8 mg twice weekly before breakfast). Lymphomas; ovarian, testicular, and breast cancer; and primary macroglobulinemia: adjust dose as peripheral count falls.

Rate of Administration

Absorption, Metabolism, Excretion
Oral absorption is adequate and reliable. Metabolism and excretion data are incomplete.

Onset, Duration of Action, $T_{1/2}$

Side Effects, Toxicity
Mild gastrointestinal upset (occasional), bone marrow depression (rapidly reversible, platelet-sparing), hepatotoxicity, exfoliative dermatitis, and allergic febrile reactions (rare).

Contraindications
Exercise care in patients with hypoplastic marrows and the "packed marrow syndrome" of chronic lymphocytic leukemia, and in those receiving concomitant radiation therapy.

Clinically Significant Drug Interactions
Allopurinol may increase the risk of bone marrow depression.

Notes

References

Cridland, M. D. Chronic lymphocytic leukemia. *Med. J. Aust.* 2:17–19, 1974.

Ezdinli, E. Z., and Stutzman, L. Chlorambucil therapy for lymphomas and chronic lymphocytic leukemia. *J. A. M. A.* 191:444–50, 1965.

Marsh, J. C., and Mitchell, M. S. Chemotherapy of cancer II. Therapy of hematologic cancers. *Drug Ther.* 4:92–109, 1974.

Masterson, J. G.; Calame, R. J.; and Nelson, J. Clinical study on the use of chlorambucil in treatment of cancer of the ovary. *Am. J. Obstet. Gynecol.* 79:1002–7, 1960.

Miller, D. G.; Diamond, H. D.; and Craver, L. F. Clinical use of chlorambucil: a critical study. *N. Engl. J. Med.* 261:525–35, 1959.

Moore, G. E.; Bross, I. D.; Ausman, R.; *et al.* The effects of chlorambucil (NSC-3088) in 374 patients with advanced cancer. Eastern clinical drug evaluation program. *Cancer Chemother. Rep.* 52:661–66, 1968.

CHLOROTRIANISENE

Trade Name
Tace®

Classification Category
Hormone (Estrogen)

Dosage Forms & Route of Administration
12-, 25-mg oral capsules

Mechanism of Action
Mode of action unknown

Indications, Dosage & Duration of Treatment
Prostate cancer: 12–25 mg/day orally.

Rate of Adminstration

Absorption, Metabolism, Excretion
Largely metabolized in the liver and excreted in the urine.

Onset, Duration of Action, $T_{1/2}$
Response to therapy is slow (6–10 weeks) and occasionally occurs after treatment is stopped.

Side Effects, Toxicity
Same as diethylstilbestrol.

Contraindications
Estrogen-sensitive carcinoma.

Clinically Significant Drug Interactions

Notes

References

CIS-DIAMMINEDICHLOROPLATINUM (CISPLATIN)

Trade Name
Platinol®, *Cis*-platinum

Classification Category
Alkylating Agent (Miscellaneous)

Dosage Forms & Route of Administration
10-mg vials; IV

Mechanism of Action
Selective inhibition of DNA synthesis; alkylating agent

Indications, Dosage & Duration of Treatment
Testicular cancer, ovarian cancer, bladder cancer, head and neck cancer: low dose 15–30 mg/M² IV daily for 5 days every three weeks; intermediate dose 30–60 mg/M² IV every week; high dose 60–120 mg/M² IV every 3 weeks.

Rate of Administration
Rapid IV infusion (15–30 minutes) for low and intermediate doses. Use slow infusion (4–8 hours) for the high dose.

Absorption, Metabolism, Excretion
Drug uptake is high in the liver, kidneys, and large and small intestines. Urinary elimination of the drug is incomplete, with only 27–43% of the drug excreted in the first 5 days. There are insufficient data to determine whether biliary or intestinal excretion takes place.

Onset, Duration of Action, $T_{1/2}$
Biphasic $T_{1/2}$: initial phase is 25–50 minutes; secondary phase is 58–73 hours. During the excretion phase, more than 90% of the drug in the blood is protein-bound.

Side Effects, Toxicity
Renal toxicity is dose-related and manifested by elevation in BUN and creatinine, hyperuricemia, and/or a decrease in creatinine clearance. Ototoxicity, nausea, vomiting, leukopenia, thrombocytopenia, anemia, anaphylactic-like reactions, peripheral neuropathies, and loss of taste may occur.

Contraindications
Impaired renal function (creatinine clearance of less than 60 ml/minute).

Clinically Significant Drug Interactions

Notes
Measures to alleviate or minimize renal toxicity include hydration, diuresis, and slow infusion.

The drug dose can be diluted in 2 liters of 5% Dextrose and 0.33–0.5 Normal Saline containing 37.5 grams of mannitol and infused over 4–8 hours. Do not administer in dextrose solution alone. The drug's stability is diminished to 2–4 hours in 5% Dextrose Injection, U.S.P. Stability can be maintained up to 24 hours in Sodium Chloride for Injection, U.S.P.

Dissolve the drug with 10 ml of Sterile Water for Injection, U.S.P. The resulting solution will contain 1 mg/ml and is stable for 20 hours at room temperature. Reconstituted solution must be stored at room temperature. Refrigerated solutions will form precipitate. Unopened vials of powder must be refrigerated.

Pretreatment hydration with 1–2 liters of fluid infused over 8–12 hours prior to dosing is recommended. Adequate hydration and urinary output must be maintained during the 24-hour period following administration. Recent studies suggesting reduced toxicities with maintained efficacy, using 24-hour infusion, need to be confirmed.

References

Earhart, R. H. Instability of *Cis*-diamminedichloroplatinum in dextrose solution. *Cancer Treat. Rep.* vol. 62, no 7. July, 1978.

Einhorn, L. H., and Donohue, J. *Cis*-diamminedichloroplatinum, vinblastine and bleomycin combination chemotherapy in disseminated testicular cancer. *Ann. Intern. Med.* 87:293–98, 1977.

Hardaker, W. T., Jr.; Stone, R. A.; and McCoy, R. Platinum nephrotoxicity. *Cancer* 34:1030–32, 1974.

Higby, D. J.; Wallace, H. J.; Albert, D. J.; and Holland, J. F. Diamminedichloroplatinum: a Phase I study showing responses in testicular and other tumors. *Cancer* 33:1219–25, 1974.

Rozencweig, M.; VonHoff, D. D.; and Muggia, F. M. Investigational chemotherapeutic agents in head and neck cancer. *Semin. Oncol.* 4:425–29, 1977.

Rozencweig, M.; VonHoff, D. D.; Slavik, M.; and Muggia, F. M. *Cis*-diamminedichloroplatinum (II). A new anticancer drug. *Ann. Intern. Med.* 86:893–912, 1977.

CYCLOPHOSPHAMIDE

Trade Name
Cytoxan®

Classification Category
Alkylating Agent (Nitrogen Mustard)

Dosage Forms & Route of Administration
25-, 50-mg oral tablets; 100-, 200-, 500-mg vials for IV administration

Mechanism of Action
Alkylating agent (cross-linking of DNA) following hepatic conversion to active metabolites by cytochrone P-450 mixed oxidase system. Subsequent activation to phosphoramide and acrolein in tissues. (See mechlorethamine monograph).

Indications, Dosage & Duration of Treatment
Beneficial effects in Hodgkin's disease and other lymphomas, multiple myeloma, chronic lymphocytic leukemia, and acute lymphoblastic leukemia. Temporary palliative effects in bronchogenic carcinoma, ovarian malignancies, cervical and breast cancers, neuroblastoma, head and neck tumors, rhabdomyosarcoma, genitourinary cancers, and soft-tissue sarcomas. Also used as an immunosuppressive agent.

Leukemia, lymphoma, and multiple myeloma: 2–3 mg/kg/day IV or PO. Continuation of therapy and maintenance dose (50–100 mg PO daily or 2 or 3 times weekly) depend on response and total leukocyte count, which should remain at 2,000–5,000/cu mm.

Lung cancer: in combination regimens administered as 500–1000 mg/M^2 IV every three weeks. (see Protocols section).

Rate of Administration
IV: infuse over 2–6 hours in 500 ml of 5% Dextrose Injection, U.S.P., to prevent hemorrhagic cystitis.

Absorption, Metabolism, Excretion
Well absorbed from gastrointestinal and parenteral sites, metabolized in the liver, and excreted by the kidneys (36–99% in 48 hours, with 30% as unchanged drug). Peak serum level is seen within 1 hour after oral administration.

Onset, Duration of Action, $T_{½}$
$T_{½}$ = 4–6 hours (IV)

Side Effects, Toxicity
Anorexia, nausea, and vomiting are common. Leukopenia (expected), thrombocytopenia, anemia (reversible), hemorrhagic colitis (isolated reports), oral mucosal ulceration and jaundice, sterile hemorrhagic cystitis (1–4%), alopecia (20–30%, reversible), dermatitis, interstitial pulmonary fibrosis, renal tubular necrosis, syndrome of inappropriate ADH, amenorrhea, azoospermia, and cardiac toxicity (with high dose) may occur.

Contraindications
Give cautiously to patients with impaired renal or hepatic function, previous x-ray therapy, previous therapy with cytotoxic agents, or bone marrow depression.

Clinically Significant Drug Interactions
Allopurinol may increase the risk of bone marrow depression. Rate of metabolism and leukopenic activity are increased with chronic high doses of microsomal enzyme inducers (e.g., phenobarbital). Inactivation may be competitively inhibited by disulfiram and chloral hydrate.

Notes
Administer the drug in the morning with ample fluid and frequent voiding to prevent the development of cytitis. Patients with any previous treatment that may have compromised the functional capacity of the bone marrow, such as x-rays or cytotoxic drugs, may require reduction of the initial loading dose by one third to one half. For IV reconstitution, add 5 ml Sterile Water for Injection, U.S.P., to 100-mg vial 20, ml to 200-mg vial, and 25 ml to 500-mg vial.

References

Boston Collaborative Drug Surveillance Program. Allopurinol and cytotoxic drugs: interaction in relation to bone marrow depression. *J. A. M. A.* 227:1026–40, 1974.

Buckner, C. D.; Rudolph, R. H.; Fefer, A.; Clift, R. A.; Epstein, R. B.; Funk, D. D.; Nelman, P. E.; Slichter, S. J.; Storb, R.; and Thomas, E. D. High-dose cyclophosphamide therapy for malignant disease. *Cancer* 29:357–65, 1972.

Coggins, P. R.; Ravdin, R. G.; Eisman, S. H. Clinical evaluation of a new alkylating agent. *Cancer* 13:1245, 1960.

Gershwin, M. E.; Goetzel, E. J.; and Steinberg, A. D. Cyclophosphamide: use in practice. *Ann. Intern. Med.* 80:531–40, 1974.

Patel, A. R.; Shah, P. C.; Rhee, H. L.; Sasson, H.; and Rao, K. P. Cyclophosphamide therapy and interstitial pulmonary fibrosis. *Cancer* 38:1542–49, 1976.

Rundles, R. W.; Lazlo, J.; Garrison, F. E., Jr.; and Hobson, J. B. The antitumor spectrum of cyclophosphamide. *Cancer Chemother. Rep.* 16:407, 1962.

Solomon, J.; Alexander, M. J.; and Steinfeld, J. L. Cyclophosphamide: a clinical study. *J. A. M. A.* 183:165–70, 1963.

CYTARABINE (CYTOSINE ARABINOSIDE)

Trade Name
Cytosar®, Ara-C

Classification Category
Antimetabolite (Pyrimidine Analogue)

Dosage Forms & Route of Administration
100-, 500-mg vials; IV, SC

Mechanism of Action
Inhibition of DNA polymerase by competition of triphosphate for deoxycytidine triphosphate.

Indications, Dosage & Duration of Treatment
Acute myelocytic (granulocytic) leukemia in adults: 100 mg/M^2 continuous IV infusion over 24 hours for 7–10 days (see Protocols section, Ara-C + Adriamycin).

Rate of Administration

Absorption, Metabolism, Excretion
The drug is metabolized rapidly by the liver and perhaps by the kidney and excreted mainly as the deaminated product. The drug is activated to Ara-CTP by phosphorylation of cytidine kinase and is inactivated by conversion to Ara-U by cytidine deaminase. After a single IV dose, the active drug is cleared from the blood in 5–20 minutes. Approximately 89–94% of the drug is excreted in the urine within 24 hours, with 5–8% excreted in the unaltered form.

Onset, Duration of Action, $T_{1/2}$
$T_{1/2}$(IV): first phase 7–17 minutes, second phase 30-200 minutes; $T_{1/2}$ (CSF) is 2 hours.

Side Effects, Toxicity
Nausea (16%), vomiting (14%), diarrhea (10%), bone marrow depression (19%), leukopenia (66%), thrombocytopenia (62%), megaloblastosis (15%), stomatitis (9%), anemia (13%), thrombophlebitis (8%), hepatic dysfunction (7%), fever (3%), abdominal pain,

esophagitis, arthralgia, and dizziness. Arachnoiditis may occur with intrathecal administration.

Contraindications
Preexisting drug-induced bone marrow suppression.

Clinically Significant Drug Interactions

Notes
The drug should not be used unless platelet and granulocyte transfusions are available.

IV: reconstitute the 100-mg vial with 5 ml Bacteriostatic Water for Injection, U.S.P., and the 500-mg vial with 10 ml Bacteriostatic Water for Injection, U.S.P. Reconstituted solutions are stable at room temperature for 48 hours. Dilute for IV infusion with Sodium Chloride for Injection, U.S.P., or 5% Dextrose Injection, U.S.P.

Mechanisms of resistance to cytarabine include reduced affinity of the triphosphate for DNA polymerase, increased intracellular deoxycitidine triphosphate, and alterations in levels of the kinase and deaminase enzymes.

References

Burke, P.J.; Serpick, A. A.; Carbone, P. P.; and Tarr, N. A clinical evaluation of dose and schedule of administration of cytosine arabinoside (NSC-63878). *Cancer Res.* 28:274-79, 1968.

Creasey, W. A.; Papac, R. J.; Markiw, M. E.; Calabresi, P.; and Welsh, A. D. Biochemical and pharmacological studies with 1-*β*-*D*-arabinofuranosyl cytosine in man, *Biochem. Pharmacol.* 15:1417–28, 1966.

Ellison, R. R.; Holland, J. F.; Weil, M.; Jacquillat, C.; Boiron, M.; Bernard, J.; Sawitsky, A.; Rosner, F.; Gussoff, B.; Silver, R. T.; Karanas, A ; Cuttner, J.; Spurr, C. L.; Hayes, D. M.; Blom, J.; Leone, L. A.; Haurani, F.; Kyle, R.; Hutchison, J. L.; Forcier, R. J.; and Moon, J. H. Arabinosyl cytosine: a useful agent in the treatment of acute leukemia in adults. *Blood* 32:507–23, 1968.

Evans, J. S.; Musser, E. A.; Mengel, G. D.; Forsbald, K. R.; and Hunter, J. H. Antitumor activity of 1-β-*D*-arabinofuranosyl cytosine hydrochloride. *Proc. Soc. Exp. Biol. Med.* 106:350, 1961.

Livingston, R. B., and Carter, S. K. Cytosine arabinoside. A clinical brochure. Part I. *Cancer Chemother. Rep.* 53:179–205, 1968.

Talley, R. W.; O'Bryan, R. M.; Tucker, W. G.; and Loo, R. V. Clinical pharmacology and human antitumor activity of cytosine arabinoside. *Cancer* 20:809–16, 1967.

Wang, J. J., and Pratt, C. G. Intrathecal arabinoside cytosine in meningeal leukemia. *Cancer* 25:531–34, 1970.

DACARBAZINE

Trade Name
DIC, DTIC®, Imidazole Carboxamide

Classification Category
Alkylating Agent (Triazene)

Dosage Forms & Route of Administration
100-, 200-mg vials; IV infusion

Mechanism of Action
Several hypotheses have been offered:

a. Inhibition of DNA synthesis by acting as a purine analogue.

b. Action as an alkylating agent by release of a mustard radical.

c. Interaction with SH groups.

Indications, Dosage & Duration of Treatment
Malignant melanoma, sarcomas, and lymphomas: the most frequently used regimens are 4.5 mg/kg/day for 10 days, to be repeated every 28 days, or 250 mg/M²/day for 5 days, to be repeated every 21 days. Single-day dosage repeated every 21 days may be as effective as 5- or 10-day courses.

Rate of Administration
Administer over 30 minutes.

Absorption, Metabolism, Excretion
Initially, the drug is found in a space greater than the extracellular fluid, and it can be detected in the CSF in low concentration (14%). The only practical route of administration is IV because of erratic oral absorption. Prior activation by cytochrone P-450 mixed oxidase system in the liver is necessary for the drug to act.

N-Demethylation in liver microsomal suspensions has been implicated as a major metabolic pathway. Thirty to 46% of the dose is excreted by a renal tubular secretory mechanism within 6 hours. Fifty percent of the drug is excreted unchanged.

Onset, Duration of Action, $T_{1/2}$

$T_{1/2}$ = 35–75 minutes for an IV dose. Residual serum levels are not detectable 24 hours after administration.

Side Effects, Toxicity

Nausea and vomiting, rare "flu-like" symptoms, rare photosensitivity, pain at infusion site, myelosuppression (leukopenia, thrombocytopenia), alopecia, facial flushing and facial paresthesias, hepatotoxicity (increased bilirubin and transaminases), and azotemia. Intractable nausea and vomiting have rarely necessitated discontinuance of DTIC®.

Contraindications

Previous hypersensitivity to the drug.

Clinically Significant Drug Interactions

Microsomal liver enzyme inducers increase the rate of metabolism of the drug.

Notes

Use lower dose in patients with impaired marrow or renal function. Store in refrigerator. Reconstitute the 100-mg and 200-mg vials with 9.9 ml and 19.7 ml Sterile Water for Injection, U.S.P., respectively, then dilute with 5% Dextrose Injection, U.S.P., or Sodium Chloride for Injection, U.S.P. Discard 12 hours after mixing. Patients may complain of burning sensation on administration.

Consider use of antiemetics.

References

Bono, V. H., Jr. Studies on the mechanism of action of DTIC (NSC-45388). *Cancer Treat. Rep.* 60:141–48, 1976.

Burke, R. J.; McCarthy, W. H.; and Milton, G. W. Imidazole carboxamide therapy in advanced malignant melanoma. *Cancer* 27:744–50, 1971.

Comis, R. L. DTIC (NSC-45388) in malignant melanoma: a perspective. *Cancer Treat. Rep.* 60:165–76, 1976.

Goldsmith, M. A.; Friedman, M. A.; and Carter, S. K. *Clinical drug data, DTIC.* National Cancer Institute, Bethesda, Maryland, 1972.

Luce, J. K.; Thurman, W. G.; Isaccs, B. L.; and Talley, R. W. Clinical trials with the antitumor agent 5-(3,3-dimethyl-1-triazeno-imidazole-4-carboxamide (NSC-45388). *Cancer Chemother. Rep.* 54:119, 1970.

DACTINOMYCIN

Trade Name
Cosmegen®, Actinomycin D

Classification Category
Natural Product (Antibiotic)

Dosage Forms & Route of Administration
0.5-mg (500-μg) ampul; IV push

Mechanism of Action
Forms stable complex with DNA and thereby inhibits DNA-dependent RNA synthesis.

Indications, Dosage & Duration of Treatment
Wilms' tumor, neuroblastoma, embryonal rhabdomyosarcoma, Ewing's sarcoma, choriocarcinoma, testicular and carcinoid tumors: usual adult dosage is 500 μg daily for a maximum of 5 days; 15 μg/kg/day for 5 days in children; course may be repeated after a 2-week rest period.

Rate of Administration
Administer through running IV infusion (5% Dextrose Injection, U.S.P., or Sodium Chloride for Injection, U.S.P.) over 10–15 minutes.

Absorption, Metabolism, Excretion
Very little active drug can be detected in the circulating blood 2 minutes after IV injection. No evidence of metabolism exists. The drug is excreted unchanged in the urine (10-20%) and bile (50%-90%) over the first 24 hours.

Onset, Duration of Action, $T_{1/2}$

Side Effects, Toxicity
Pain on local infiltration (skin necrosis), nausea, and vomiting in patients 2 hours after administration; occasional cramps and diarrhea, bone marrow depression, stomatitis, erythema, hyperpigmentation, with occasional desquamation in areas of previous irradiation; and acne.

Contraindications

Clinically Significant Drug Interactions

Notes

Use with care in liver disease and in presence of inadequate marrow function.

Prophylactic antiemetics are helpful.

Hematopoietic, renal, and hepatic functions should be monitored. Leukocyte counts should be taken daily and platelet counts taken every 3 days during therapy.

Reconstitute with 1.1 ml Sterile Water for Injection, U.S.P., administer IV push. Avoid extravasation.

Store at room temperature. Use immediately after mixing.

References

Burgert, E.O., and Glidewell, O. Dactinomycin in Wilms' tumor. *J. A. M. A.* 199:464–68, 1967.

Farber, S.; D'Angio, G. T.; Evan, A. D.; and Mitus, A. Clinical studies of actinomycin D with special reference to Wilms' tumor in children. *Ann. N. Y. Acad. Sci.* 89:421–25, 1960.

Reich, E. Biochemistry of actinomycins. *Cancer Res.* 23:1428–41, 1963.

Waksman, S. A., ed. The actinomycins and their importance in the treatment of tumors in animals and man: introduction. *Ann. N. Y. Acad. Sci.* 89:285–86, 1960.

DAUNORUBICIN

Trade Name
(Investigational NSC-82151), Daunomycin, Rubidomycin, Cerutidine®

Classification Category
Natural Product (Antibiotic)

Dosage Forms & Route of Administration
20-mg vials; IV push, IV infusion

Mechanism of Action
Binds to nucleic acids by intercalating between base pairs, thus inhibiting RNA synthesis by steric disordering of the DNA template.

Indications, Dosage & Duration of Treatment
Acute myelocytic and lymphocytic leukemia: 1 mg/kg/day IV for 5 days or 60 mg/M²/day IV for 3 days; repeat at 3–6 week intervals.

Rate of Administration
Administer through running IV infusion.

Absorption, Metabolism, Excretion
Total output of the drug and its metabolites in the urine is low. There is probably significant biliary excretion of the drug. Hepatic metabolism may occur.

Onset, Duration of Action, $T_{1/2}$
Plasma $T_{1/2}$ is biphasic: initial phase is 1 hour; secondary phase is 17 hours.

Side Effects, Toxicity
Leukopenia (65%), thrombocytopenia (54%), anemia (5%), cardiotoxicity (2%), nausea (22%), vomiting (37%), diarrhea (25%), mucositis (15%), fever (33%), phlebitis (30%), skin rash (6%), alopecia (35%), and renal tubular damage. Cardiac toxicity is dose-related (e.g., greater than 600 mg/M² total dose).

Contraindications
Preexisting drug-induced bone marrow suppression, hepatic dysfunction, active congestive heart failure, and previous therapy with adriamycin at or above a total dose of 550 mg/M².

Clinically Significant Drug Interactions

Notes

Follow for EKG abnormalities and signs of heart failure.

Colors urine red (not hematuria).

Consider use of antiemetics.

Store at room temperature. Reconstitute with 5–10 ml Sterile Water for Injection, U.S.P. Discard 6 hours after mixing.

Necrosis may occur with extravasation.

References

Alberts, D. S.; Beachur, N. R.; and Holtzman, J. L. The pharmacokinetics of daunomycin in man. *Clin. Pharm. Therap.* 12:96–104, 1971.

Boiron, M.; Jacquillat, C.; Weil, M.; Tanzer, J.; Levy, D.; Sultan, C.; and Bernard, J. Daunorubicin in the treatment of acute myelocytic leukemia. *Lancet* 1:330–33, 1969.

DiMarco, A.; Gaetani, M.; Dorigotti, L.; Soldati, M.; and Bellini, O. Experimental studies on the antitumor activity of daunomycin: a new antibiotic with antitumor activity. *Tumori* 49:203–17, 1963.

Livingston, R. B., and Carter, S. K. *Daunomycin: a chemotherapy fact sheet of the National Cancer Institute.* Bethesda, Maryland, 1970.

Samuels, L.D.; Newton, W. A., Jr.; and Heyn, R. Daunorubicin therapy in advanced neuroblastoma. *Cancer* 27:831–34, 1971.

Tarr, C.; Tasaka, H.; Yu, K-P; Murphy, M. L.; and Karrolsky, D. A. Daunomycin: an antitumor antibiotic in the treatment of neoplastic disease. *Cancer* 20:333–53, 1967.

Weil, M.; Glidewell, O. J.; Jacquillat, C.; Leuy, R.; Serpick, A.; Wiernik, P.; Cuttner, J.; Hoogstraten, B.; Wasserman, L.; Ellison, R.; Gailini, S.; Brunner, K.; Silver, R.; Rege, V.; Cooper, M.; Lowenstein, L.; Nissen, N.; Haurani, F.; Blom, J.; Boiron, M.; Bernard, J.; and Holland, J. Daunorubicin in the therapy of acute granolocytic leukemia. *Cancer Res.* 33:921–28, 1973.

VonHoff, D. D., and Slavik, M. *Daunomycin (NSC-82151).* Clinical Brochure. National Cancer Institute, Bethesda, Maryland, 1976.

DIETHYLSTILBESTROL

Trade Name
Diethylstilbestrol®, DES®

Classification Category
Hormone (Nonsteroidal Estrogen)

Dosage Forms & Route of Administration
0.1-, 0.25-, 0.5-, 1-, 5-, 10-, 25-, 50-, 100-mg oral tablets

Mechanism of Action
The postulated mode of action is direct antitumor activity and inhibition of pituitary production of prolactin and gonadotropin.

Indications, Dosage & Duration of Treatment
Carcinoma of the prostate: 1–3 mg/day orally.

Postmenopausal breast cancer: up to 15 mg/day orally in divided doses for a minimum of 3 months.

Rate of Administration

Absorption, Metabolism, Excretion
Largely metabolized in the liver and excreted in the urine.

Onset, Duration of Action, $T_{1/2}$
Response to therapy is slow (6–10 weeks) and occasionally occurs after treatment is stopped (withdrawal response).

Side Effects, Toxicity
Nausea (20%), which may disappear after 3 weeks; vomiting with large doses; fluid retention (older patients should be placed on low salt diet and possibly diuretics); gynecomastia in men, and breast tenderness in women. Lower extremity edema, without congestive heart failure, is common. High doses have been implicated in increased cardiovascular and cerebrovascular deaths in men with cancer of the prostate.

Contraindications

Known or suspected cancer of the breast, except in selected patients. Estrogen-dependent neoplasia, pregnancy, abnormal genital bleeding, active or past history of thrombophlebitis.

Clinically Significant Drug Interactions

Notes

Use in low doses in men with prostate cancer. Use in postmenopausal breast cancer patients only (30% response) or in women with known positive estrogen receptors (60% response). Serum calcium can rise rapidly in 5–10% of the breast cancer patients, especially in those with bone disease. Stop DES therapy if serum calcium is over 13.0 milligrams percent. Edema may occur with poor cardiac function. Palliative in patients with advanced prostatic cancer, often in conjunction with orchiectomy (orchiectomy appears to be as effective as estrogen therapy, with fewer side effects and longer periods of survival).

Monitor serum calcium levels frequently during first 2 weeks of treatment in women with bone metastases.

Symptoms of hypercalcemia include increased thirst, polyuria, drowsiness, and constipation.

References

Bailar, J. C., and Byar, D. P. Veterans Administration Cooperative Urological Research Group. Estrogen treatment for cancer of the prostate: early results with 3 doses of diethylstilbestrol and placebo. *Cancer* 26:257–61, 1970.

Carter, A. C.; Sedransk, N.; Kelley, R. M.; Ansfield, F. J.; Ravdin, R. G.; Talley, R. W.; and Potter, N. R. Diethylstilbestrol: recommended dosages for different categories of breast cancer patients. Report of the Cooperative Breast Cancer Group. *J. A. M. A.* 237:2079–85, 1977.

Haddow, A.; Watkinson, J. M.; and Paterson, E. Influences of synthetic oestrogens upon advanced malignant disease. *Brit. Med. J.* 2:393–408, 1944.

Kennedy, B. J. Hormonal therapies in breast cancer. *Semin. Oncol.* 1:119–30, 1974.

DOXORUBICIN

Trade Name
Adriamycin®

Classification Category
Natural Product (Antibiotic)

Dosage Forms & Route of Administration
10-, 50-mg vials; IV push, IV infusion

Mechanism of Action
Alters DNA and inhibits RNA synthesis by intercalating into DNA.

Indications, Dosage & Duration of Treatment
Acute lymphoblastic leukemia, acute myelocytic leukemia, lymphomas, sarcomas, and carcinoma of the bladder, breast, thyroid, and lung: 50 mg/M^2/day IV every 21 days in combination therapy (see Protocols section).

Rate of Administration
Administer by IV push or IV infusion over 30 minutes.

Absorption, Metabolism, Excretion
Hepatic clearance is approximately 60% of hepatic blood flow. Approximately 4–5% of the administered dose is excreted in the urine in 5 days. Forty to 50% of the administered dose is recovered in the bile or feces in 7 days.

Onset, Duration of Action, $T_{1/2}$
Biphasic $T_{1/2}$: initial phase is 1 hour; secondary phase is 17 hours.

Side Effects, Toxicity
Nausea and vomiting (46%), fever (5%), local phlebitis, necrosis if extravasated, bone marrow depression (74%), alopecia (100%), cardiac toxicity related to cumulative dose, and stomatitis (15%).

Contraindications
Avoid giving to patients with clinical congestive heart failure. Reduce the dose in patients with liver failure and preexisting myelosuppression.

Clinically Significant Drug Interactions

Notes

Monitor for EKG abnormalities and signs of heart failure. Two types of cardiotoxicity may occur: acute transient reversible electrocardiographic alterations; and a total dose-dependent irreversible syndrome of congestive heart failure, which may be unresponsive to cardiac supportive therapy. Doxorubicin is less cardiotoxic than daunorubicin in a given myelosuppressive dose.

Store at room temperature. Reconstitute the 10-mg and 50-mg vials with 5 ml and 25 ml of Sodium Chloride for Injection, U.S.P., respectively. The reconstituted solution is stable for 24 hours at room temperature. Discard any unused portion. Avoid extravasation.

Plasma $T_{1/2}$ is elevated and prolonged in patients with hepatic dysfunction. Reduce dose by 50% for a bilirubin >1.5 mg/dl and 75% for a bilirubin >3.0 mg/dl.

Total cumulative dose should be limited to a maximum of 550 mg/M^2.

May color urine red.

References

Benjamin, R. F.; Riggs, C. E., Jr.; and Bachur, N. R. Pharmacokinetics and metabolism of Adriamycin in man. *Clin. Pharmacol. Ther.* 14:592–600, 1973.

Blum, R. H.; and Carter, S. K. Adriamycin, a new anticancer drug with significant clinical activity. *Ann. Intern. Med.* 80:249–52, 1974.

Bonadonna, G.; Monfardini, S.; deLena, M.; and Fossati-Bellani, F. Clinical evaluation of Adriamycin, a new antitumor antibiotic. *Brit. Med. J.* 3:503–6, 1969.

DiFronzo, G.; Lenaz, L.; and Bonadonna, G. Distribution and excretion of Adriamycin in man. *Biomedicine* 19:169-71, 1973.

Lenaz, L., and Page, J. A. Cardiotoxicity of Adriamycin and related anthracyclines. *Cancer Treat. Rev.* 3:111–20, 1976.

Smith, I. E., and McElwain, T. J. Letter: Adriamycin in acute leukaemia. *Lancet* 2:161, 1974.

5-FLUOROURACIL

Trade Name
Fluorouracil®, 5-Fluorouracil, 5–FU

Classification Category
Antimetabolite (Pyrimidine Analogue)

Dosage Forms & Route of Administration
500-mg ampul; IV administration

Mechanism of Action
The uracil analogue is converted intracellularly to FdUMP, which binds to thymidylate synthetase and inhibits subsequent DNA synthesis. It is also thought to produce a fraudulent RNA and to block uracil phosphatase, thereby inhibiting utilization of preformed uracil in RNA synthesis.

Indications, Dosage & Duration of Treatment
Carcinoma of the colon, metastatic breast carcinoma, and carcinoma of the stomach and pancreas (see Protocols section for combination therapy).

The dose when used as a single agent is 10-15 mg/kg/week in a single IV injection. This may be preceded by a 5-day loading course. Hepatic artery infusion produces high hepatic drug concentration with minimal systemic toxicity.

Rate of Administration
IV push.

Absorption, Metabolism, Excretion
The drug is metabolized in the liver and excreted as respiratory carbon dioxide, urea, and several other substances in the urine. Following a single IV dose, 15% of the drug is excreted unchanged within 6 hours; 90% of this amount is excreted in the first hour. It distributes in a volume equal to the total body water and readily enters CSF and effusions.

Onset, Duration of Action, $T_{1/2}$
$T_{1/2}$ = 10–20 minutes after IV administration.

Side Effects, Toxicity
Nausea and vomiting, anorexia, bone marrow depression (nadir at 10–14 days), leukopenia, thrombocytopenia, anemia, maculopapular rash, alopecia, increased skin pigmentation, and cerebellar ataxia (5%). Stomatitis and diarrhea are early signs of drug toxicity and usually necessitate discontinuing the drug.

Contraindications
Poor nutritional state and preexisting bone marrow depression.

Clinically Significant Drug Interactions

Notes
Exposure to strong sunlight may intensify skin reactions. Decrease dose in patients with diminished liver, renal, or bone marrow function.

References

Brennan, M. J., and Vaitkevicius, V. K. 5-Fluorouracil in clinical cancer experience with 155 patients. *Cancer Chemother. Rep.* 6:8–11, 1960.

Curreri, A. R.; Ansfield, F. J.; and McIver, F. Clinical studies with 5-fluorouracil. *Cancer Res.* 18:478–84, 1958.

Douglass, H. O.; and Mittleman, A. Metabolic studies of 5-fluorouracil. II. Influence of the route of administration on the dynamics of distribution in man. *Cancer* 34:1878–81, 1974.

Hahn, R. G.; Moertel, C. G.; Shutt, A. J.; and Bruckner, H. W. A double-blind comparison of intensive course 5-fluorouracil by oral vs. intravenous route in the treatment of colorectal carcinoma. *Cancer* 35:1031–35, 1975.

Heidelberger, C., and Ansfield, F. J. Experimental and clinical use of fluorinated pyrimidines in cancer chemotherapy. *Cancer Res.* 23:1226–43, 1963.

Horton, J.; Olson, K. B.; Sullivan, J.; Reilly, C.; Shnider, B.; and the Eastern Cooperative Oncology Group. 5-Fluorouracil in cancer: an improved regimen. *Ann. Intern. Med.* 73:897–900, 1970.

Jacobs, E. M.; Luce, J. K.; and Wood, D. A. Treatment of cancer with weekly intravenous 5-fluorouracil. *Cancer* 22:1233–38, 1968.

FLUOXYMESTERONE

Trade Name
Halotestin®

Classification Category
Hormone (Androgen)

Dosage Forms & Route of Administration
2-, 5-, 10-mg oral tablets

Mechanism of Action

Indications, Dosage & Duration of Treatment
Palliation of androgen-responsive, advanced, female breast cancer: 15–30 mg daily in divided doses.

Rate of Administration

Absorption, Metabolism, Excretion
The drug is rapidly absorbed, and is accumulated and conjugated in the liver and to some extent in the kidney. It is rapidly eliminated by glomerular filtration and tubular secretion.

Onset, Duration of Action, $T_{1/2}$
Response is slow (8–12 weeks).

Side Effects, Toxicity
Virilizing effects, nausea and vomiting, fluid retention, hypercalcemia, and liver function abnormalities with rare cholestatic jaundice.

Contraindications
Carcinoma of the male breast or prostate; cardiac, hepatic, or renal decompensation; and hypercalcemia.

Clinically Significant Drug Interactions

Notes

Frequent plasma calcium determinations are recommened.

Cautiously reinstitute therapy after correction of hypercalcemia.

References

Kennedy, B. J. Hormonal therapies in breast cancer. *Semin. Oncol.* 1:119–30, 1974.

HEXAMETHYLMELAMINE

Trade Name
(Investigational NSC-13875)

Classification Category
Miscellaneous Agent

Dosage Forms & Route of Administration
50-, 100-mg capsules

Mechanism of Action
It has been postulated that the drug inhibits RNA and DNA synthesis by means of an antimetabolite pathway.

Indications, Dosage & Duration of Treatment
Cancer of the ovary: The drug is possibly indicated in patients who have become refractory to therapy with alkylating agents, or in patients in whom therapy with alkylating agents is contraindicated. Dosage when used as a single agent: 8 mg/kg/day (300 mg/M^2) continuously or as tolerated. Intermittent regimen: 21 days (8 mg/kg/day) on and 21 days off the drug. This regimen may be better tolerated and may be required if gastrointestinal toxicity or neurotoxicity becomes severe.

Rate of Administration

Absorption, Metabolism, Excretion
When the drug is administered orally, the peak plasma level is reached in 1 hour. It is rapidly N-demethylated in the body, probably by the liver. The drug is excreted as metabolites in the urine, with no significant amount of the drug found in the feces.

Onset, Duration of Action, $T_{1/2}$
$T_{1/2} = 13$ hours

Side Effects, Toxicity
Gastrointestinal: nausea, vomiting, and anorexia (54%). Hematologic: leukopenia $<2{,}000/mm^3$ and thrombocytopenia $<75{,}000/mm^3$ (8%). CNS: paresthesia, numbness, sleep disturbance, hallucinations (3%),

and depression; questionable seizure and Parkinson-like syndrome with ataxia (3%). Dermatologic: skin rashes, pruritus, eczematous skin lesions (3%), and alopecia (1%).

Contraindications
Therapy with the drug should be deferred for at least 3 weeks after prior therapy with an alkylating agent.

Clinically Significant Drug Interactions

Notes

References

Bergevin, P. R., Tormey, D. C.; and Blom, J. Clinical evaluation of hexamethylmelamine (NSC-13875). *Cancer Chemother. Rep.* 57:51–58, 1973.

Legha, S. S.; Slavik, M.; and Carter, S. K. Hexamethylmelamine: an evaluation of its role in the therapy of cancer. *Cancer* 38:27–35, 1976.

National Cancer Institute. *Guideline for the clinical use of hexamethylmelamine (NSC-13875).* Bethesda, Maryland, 1977.

Worzalla, J. F.; Ramirez, G.; and Bryan, G. T. N-demethylation of the antineoplastic agent hexamethylmelamine by rats and man. *Cancer Res.* 33:2810–15, 1973.

HYDROXYUREA

Trade Name
Hydrea®

Classification Category
Miscellaneous Agent (Substituted Urea)

Dosage Forms & Route of Administration
500-mg oral capsule

Mechanism of Action
Inhibits ribonucleotide reductase, preventing conversion of ribo to deoxyribonucleotides, and subsequent DNA synthesis.

Indications, Dosage & Duration of Treatment
Chronic myelocytic leukemia, melanoma, recurrent metastatic or inoperable ovarian carcinoma: 20–30 mg/kg/day as a single dose. In patients with acute leukemia or blastic crisis of chronic myeloblastic leukemia, 50 mg/kg/day will reliably lower very high white blood cell counts within 24–48 hours.

Rate of Administration

Absorption, Metabolism, Excretion
The drug is readily absorbed from the gastrointestinal tract. One-half of the dose is degraded by the liver and excreted as respiratory carbon dioxide and as urea. The remaining portion is excreted intact in the urine.

Onset, Duration of Action, $T_{1/2}$
Peak serum concentrations are attained within 2 hours. Levels decline rapidly and there is no cumulative effect with repeated administration. The drug passes the blood-brain barrier. CSF concentrations are attained within 3 hours with oral administration.

Side Effects, Toxicity
Anorexia, nausea and vomiting, drowsiness, bone marrow depression, megaloblastic anemia (usually self-limiting), and dermatological reactions. Stomatitis, diarrhea, and alopecia are less common.

Contraindications
Marked bone marrow depression or severe anemia. The drug may have teratogenic effects.

Clinically Significant Drug Interactions

Notes
Decrease the dose in patients with bone marrow and renal dysfunction.

Higher blood levels are obtained if the drug is given in a large, single oral dose.

Recovery from bone marrow depression is usually rapid when drug therapy is interrupted.

Bone marrow studies should be done prior to and periodically during therapy. Complete blood count, including hemoglobin, total leukocyte counts, and platelet counts, should be performed at least weekly during therapy.

The contents of a capsule may be dissolved in water for easier oral administration.

References

Dethlefsen, L. A., and Riley, R. M. Hydroxyurea effects in the C3H mouse. II. Mammary tumor cell kinetics. *Cell Tissue Kinet.* 6:173–84, 1973.

Fishbein, W. N.; Carbone, P. P.; Freireich, E. J.; Misra, W. N.; and Frei, E. Clinical trials of hydroxyurea in patients with cancer and leukemia. *Clin. Pharmacol. Therap.* 5:574–80, 1964.

Kennedy, B. J. Hydroxyurea in chronic myelogenous leukemia. *Ann. Intern. Med.* 70:1084–85, 1969.

Kennedy, B. J., and Yarbro, J. W. Metabolic and therapeutic effects of hydroxyurea in chronic myeloid leukemia. *J. A. M. A.* 195:1038–43, 1966.

Krakoff, I. H.; Brown, N. C.; and Reichard, P. Inhibition of ribonucleoside diphosphate reductase by hydroxyurea. *Cancer Res.* 28:1559–65, 1968.

Lerner, H. J.; Beckloff, G. J.; and Godwin, M. C. Hydroxyurea (NSC-32065): intermittent therapy in malignant diseases. *Cancer Chemother. Rep.* 53:385–95, 1969.

LOMUSTINE (CCNU)

Trade Name
CeeNU®

Classification Category
Alkylating Agent (Nitrosourea)

Dosage Forms & Route of Administration
10-, 40-, 100-mg oral capsules

Mechanism of Action
Alkylating agent (not firmly established)

Indications, Dosage & Duration of Treatment
Brain tumors, both primary and metastatic, and as a secondary therapy for Hodgkin's disease: 130 mg/M^2 as a single oral dose every 6 weeks. In individuals with compromised bone marrow function, reduce the dose to 100 mg/M^2 every 6 weeks.

Rate of Administration

Absorption, Metabolism, Excretion
The drug is rapidly absorbed, degraded, and slowly excreted in the urine (50% in 12 hours and 75% in 4 days). Peak plasma concentration of metabolites is reached in 1–6 hours. The CSF levels of metabolites are 15–50% higher than concurrent plasma levels of metabolites. Some enterohepatic circulation probably occurs.

Onset, Duration of Action, $T_{1/2}$
Biphasic $T_{1/2}$: initial phase is 6 hours; secondary phase is 1 to 2 days.

Side Effects, Toxicity
Nausea and vomiting, stomatitis, alopecia, renal toxicity, hepatotoxicity (reversible), and impaired bone marrow function (delayed for 3–6 weeks after administration).

Contraindications
Previous hypersensitivity to the drug.

Clinically Significant Drug Interactions

Notes

Use antiemetics for nausea and vomiting. Reduce dosage of CCNU for patients with impaired marrow function. Store in refrigerator (stable for 1 year). Take with fluids on empty stomach.

Periodic monitoring of renal, hepatic, and bone marrow functions is recommended.

References

Hansen, H. H.; Selawry, O. S.; Muggia, F. M.; and Walker, M. D. Clinical studies with 1-(2-chloroethyl)-3-cyclohexyl-1-nitrosourea (NSC-79037). *Cancer Res.* 31:23–27, 1971.

Hoogstraten, B.; Gottlieb, J. A.; Caoili, E.; Tucker, W. G.; Talley, R. W.; and Hallt, H. CCNU [1-(2-chloroethyl)-3-cyclohexyl-1-nitrosourea, NSC-79037] in the treatment of cancer. Phase II study. *Cancer* 32:38–43, 1973.

Sponzo, R. W.; DeVita, V. T.; and Oliverio, V. T. Physiologic disposition of 1-(2-chloroethyl)-3-(4-methyl cyclohexyl)-1-nitrosourea (MeCCNU) in man. *Cancer* 31:1154–59, 1973.

Wasserman, T. H.; Slavik, M.; and Carter, S. K. Review of CCNU in clinical cancer therapy. *Cancer Treat. Rev.* 1:131–51, 1974.

Wasserman, T. H.; Slavik, M.; and Carter, S. K. Clinical comparison of the nitrosoureas. *Cancer* 36:1258–68, 1975.

MECHLORETHAMINE

Trade Name
Mustargen®

Classification Category
Alkylating Agent (Nitrogen Mustard)

Dosage Forms & Route of Administration
10-mg vial; IV

Mechanism of Action
Alkylating agents react by contributing an unstable electrophilic alkyl group ($R\text{-}CH_2$) through covalent bond formation with organic and inorganic ions within the cell. Most agents are bifunctional and are able to cross-link 2 molecules of nucleoprotein, thereby inhibiting replication and transcription. DNA miscoding and breakage may also occur.

Indications, Dosage & Duration of Treatment
Disseminated Hodgkin's disease, other lymphomas and myeloproliferative diseases, and palliation of cancer of the lung: 0.4 mg/kg; dose may be given as a single injection (preferred) or divided (see Protocols section for combination therapy).

Rate of Administration
IV push into rapidly flowing IV infusion (5% Dextrose Injection, U.S.P., or Sodium Chloride for Injection, U.S.P.).

Absorption, Metabolism, Excretion
Rapid biotransformation with no opportunity for renal excretion. Ninety percent of the drug is cleared from the blood in 1 minute and 50% appears in the urine in 24 hours.

Onset, Duration of Action, $T_{1/2}$

Side Effects, Toxicity
Nausea and vomiting (may last 24 hours), thrombophlebitis, granulocytopenia and thrombocytopenia (maximal 2 to 3 weeks after injection), stomatitis, maculopapular skin eruption, herpes zoster,

amenorrhea, azoospermia, thrombosis, bone marrow depression, tinnitis, vertigo, and hearing loss.

Contraindications
Foci of acute or chronic suppurative inflammation and infectious granuloma.

Clinically Significant Drug Interactions

Notes
Nausea and vomiting may be minimized by giving antiemetics 30 minutes before use.

If contact with skin or mucous membranes occurs, wash with water or 2% sodium thiosulfate (use of rubber gloves advised). For extravasation, infiltrate with either Sodium Chloride for Injection, U.S.P., or 1/6 molar sodium thiosulfate. (To prepare 1/6 molar sodium solution, dilute 4 ml of 10% sodium thiosulfate injection with 6 ml of Sterile Water for Injection, U.S.P.)

Reconstitute immediately prior to use with 10 ml of Sterile Water for Injection, U.S.P.

References

Daneshek, W.; Weisfuse, L.; and Stein, L. Nitrogen mustard therapy in Hodgkin's disease. *Blood* 4:328, 1949.

Gilman, A. The initial clinical trial of nitrogen mustard. *Am. J. Surg.* 105:574–78, 1963.

Gold, G. L.; Schnider, B. I.; Salvin, L. G.; Schneiderman, M. A.; Colsky, J.; Owens, A. H., Jr.; Krant, M. J.; Miller, S. P.; Frei, E., III; Hall, T. C.; Spurr, C. L.; McIntyre, O. R.; Hoogstraten, B.; and Holland, J. F. The use of mechlorethamine, cyclophosphamide, and uracil mustard in neoplastic disease: a cooperative study. *J. Clin. Pharmacol. New Drugs* 10:110–20, 1970.

Karnofsky, D. A. Nitrogen mustards in the treatment of neoplastic disease. *Adv. Intern. Med.* 4:1, 1950.

Rutman, R. J.; Chun, E. H.; and Jones, J. Observations on the mechanism of the alkylation reaction between nitrogen mustard and DNA. *Biochem. Biophys. Acta* 174:663–73, 1969.

Slack, N.H. Bronchogenic carcinoma: nitrogen mustard as a surgical adjuvant and factors influencing survival. University Surgical Adjuvant Lung Project. *Cancer* 25:987–1002, 1970.

Warwick, G. P. The mechanism of action of alkylating agents. *Cancer Res.* 23:1315–33, 1963.

MEDROXYPROGESTERONE ACETATE

Trade Name
Provera®, Depo-Provera®

Classification Category
Hormone (Progestin)

Dosage Forms & Route of Administration
2.5-, 10-mg oral tablets; 50 mg/ml IM suspension

Mechanism of Action

Indications, Dosage & Duration of Treatment
Carcinoma of the kidney, breast, and endometrium: 400–800 mg/week IM or PO.

Rate of Administration

Absorption, Metabolism, Excretion
The drug is metabolized in the liver and excreted to some extent in the urine.

Onset, Duration of Action, $T_{1/2}$

Side Effects, Toxicity
Gastrointestinal disturbances, fluid retention, headache, dizziness, oligomenorrhea or amenorrhea, congestion of the breast, decreased libido, and occasional liver function abnormalities.

Contraindications

Clinically Significant Drug Interactions

Notes

Use with care in presence of liver dysfunction.

Oral doses of 300 mg daily yield results approximately equal to those obtained by the IM route, but high-dose oral tablets are not commercially available.

References

Anderson, D. G. Management of advanced endometrial adenocarcinoma with medroxyprogesterone acetate. *Am. J. Obstet. Gynecol.* 92:87–99, 1965.

Kennedy, B. J. Hormone therapy for advanced breast cancer. *Cancer* 18:1551–57, 1965.

Muggia, F. M.; Cassileth, P. A.; Ochoa, M.; Flatow, F. A.; Gellhorn, A.; and Hyman, G. A. Treatment of breast cancer with medroxyprogesterone acetate. *Ann. Intern. Med.* 68:328–37, 1968.

Samuels, M. L.; Sullivan, P.; and Howe, C. D. Medroxyprogesterone acetate in the treatment of renal cell carcinoma (hypernephroma). *Cancer* 22:525–32, 1968.

Stoll, B. A. *Endocrine therapy in malignant disease.* Philadelphia: W. B. Saunders Company, 1972.

Segaloff, A. Hormonal therapy of breast cancer. *Cancer* 30:1541–42, 1972.

MEGESTROL ACETATE

Trade Name
Megace®

Classification Category
Hormone (Progestin)

Dosage Forms & Route of Administration
20-, 40-mg oral tablets

Mechanism of Action

Indications, Dosage & Duration of Treatment
Palliative treatment of carcinoma of the kidney, breast (160 mg/day in divided doses), and endometrium (40–320 mg/day in divided doses).

Rate of Administration

Absorption, Metabolism, Excretion
The drug is metabolized in the liver and excreted to some extent in the urine.

Onset, Duration of Action, $T_{1/2}$

Side Effects, Toxicity
Thrombophlebitis, fluid retention

Contraindications

Clinically Significant Drug Interactions

Notes

Use with caution in patients with a history of thrombophlebitis.

Adequate clinical trial usually requires 2 months of continuous treatment.

References

Bloom, H. J. G.; Roe, F. J.; and Matchley, B. C. V. Sex hormones and renal neoplasia. *Cancer* 20:2118–24, 1967.

Kennedy, B. J. A progestogen for treatment of advanced endometrial cancer. *J. A. M. A.* 184:758–61, 1963.

Kistner, R. W.; Griffiths, C. T.; and Craig, J. M. Use of progestational agents in the management of endometrial cancer. *Cancer* 18:1563–79, 1965.

Talley, R. W.; Moorhead, E. L.,; Tucker, W. G.; San Diego, E. L.; and Brennan, M. J. Treatment of metastatic hypernephroma. *J. A. M. A.* 207:322–28, 1969.

Wait, R. B. Megestrol acetate in the management of advanced endometrial carcinoma. *Obst. Gynecol.* 41:129–36, 1973.

MELPHALAN

Trade Name
Alkeran®

Classification Category
Alkylating Agent (Nitrogen Mustard)

Dosage Forms & Route of Administration
2-mg oral tablets

Mechanism of Action
Alkylating agent (cross-linking of DNA). (See Mechlorethamine Drug Monograph).

Indications, Dosage & Duration of Treatment
Multiple myeloma: administered in either intermittent high-dose courses (0.25 mg/kg/day for 4 days, to be repeated every 6 weeks) or low-dose continuous regimen (6 mg/day) adjusted on the basis of blood counts done at weekly intervals. Various other dosage regimens are discussed in the literature. Probably active in ovarian, breast, and testicular carcinoma.

Rate of Administration

Absorption, Metabolism, Excretion
The drug is well absorbed orally, active in the blood for 6 hours, and metabolized slowly.

Onset, Duration of Action, $T_{1/2}$

Side Effects, Toxicity
Nausea and vomiting (infrequent); and dose-related, bone marrow depression, producing anemia, neutropenia, and thrombocytopenia.

Contraindications

Clinically Significant Drug Interactions

Notes

If the leukocyte count falls below 3,000 cells/cu mm or the platelet count below 100,000/cu mm, the drug should be discontinued until the blood elements have had a chance to recover.

References

Bergsagel, D. E. Treatment of plasma cell myeloma. *Brit. J. Haematol.* 33:443–49, 1976.

Bergsagel, D. E. Plasma cell myeloma. *Drug Ther.* 6:72–81, 1976.

Bergsagel, D. E.; Sprague, C. C.; Austin, C.; and Griffith, K. M. Evaluation of new chemotherapeutic agents in the treatment of multiple myeloma. IV. L-Phenylalanine mustard (NSC-8806). *Cancer Chemother. Rep.* 21:87, 1962.

Fisher, B.; Carbone, P.; Economu, S. G.; Frelick, R.; Glass, A.; Lerner, H.; Redmond, C.; Zelen, M.; Band, P.; Katrych, D. L.; Wolmark, N.; and Fisher, E. R. L-phenylalanine mustard (L-PAM) in the management of primary breast cancer. *N. Engl. J. Med.* 292:117–22, 1975.

Frick, H. C.; Tretter, P.; Tretter, W.; and Hyman, G. A. Disseminated carcinoma of the ovary treated by L-phenylalanine mustard. *Cancer* 21:508–13, 1968.

Hoogstraten, B.; Sheehe, P.R.; Cuttner, J.; Cooper, T.; Kyle, R. A.; Oberfield, R. A.; Townsend, S. R.; Harley, J. B.; Hayes, D. M.; Costa, G.; and Holland, J. F. Melphalan in multiple myeloma. *Blood* 30:74–83, 1967.

6-MERCAPTOPURINE

Trade Name
Purinethol®, 6-mercaptopurine, 6-MP

Classification Category
Antimetabolite (Purine Analogue)

Dosage Forms & Route of Administration
50-mg oral tablets

Mechanism of Action
Antimetabolite (purine antagonist), inhibiting RNA and DNA synthesis. Intracellular conversion to 6-thioinosinic acid, which may suppress *de novo* purine biosynthesis, purine salvage pathways, and interconversion reactions, resulting in depletion of purine pools.

Indications, Dosage & Duration of Treatment
Acute myelocytic leukemia: 2.5 mg/kg/day in a single dose until bone marrow remission occurs. Also active in acute lymphocytic and chronic myelogenous leukemia. Usually used in combination therapy.

Rate of Administration

Absorption, Metabolism, Excretion
Rapid oral absorption occurs, and maximum serum levels are attained within 2 hours. The drug is rapidly metabolized by the liver and excreted by the kidneys (46% in 24 hours).

Onset, Duration of Action, $T_{1/2}$

Side Effects, Toxicity
Anorexia, nausea, vomiting, gastrointestinal ulceration, skin eruptions, bone marrow depression, reversible cholestatic jaundice, hepatic necrosis, dermatitis, and drug fever.

Contraindications

Clinically Significant Drug Interactions
Allopurinol inhibits metabolism of the drug by xanthine oxidase.

Notes
Reduce dosage to about 25% of the standard dose in patients receiving allopurinol concurrently.

References

Boston Collaborative Drug Surveillance Program: Allopurinol and cytotoxic drugs . . . interaction in relation to bone marrow depression. *J. A. M. A.* 227:1026–40, 1974.

Burchenal, J. H.; Murphy, M. L.; Ellison, R. R.; Sykes, M. P.; Tan, C. T.; Leone, L. A.; Karnovsky, D. A.; Carver, L. F.; Dargeon, H. W.; and Rhoads, C. P. Clinical evaluation of a new antimetabolite, 6-mercaptopurine, in the treatment of leukemia and allied diseases. *Blood* 8:965–99, 1953.

Elison, G. B. Biochemistry and pharmacology of purine analogs. *Fed. Proc.* 26:898–904, 1967.

Hyman, G. H.; Gellhorn, A.; and Wolff, J. A. The therapeutic effect of mercaptopurine in a variety of human neoplastic diseases. *Ann. N. Y. Acad. Sci.* 60:430, 1954.

Shorey, J.; Schouker, S.; Suki, W. N.; and Combes, B. Hepatoxicity of mercaptopurine. *Arch. Intern. Med.* 122:54–58, 1968.

METHOTREXATE

Trade Name
Methotrexate®, MTX

Classification Category
Antimetabolite (Folic Acid Analogue)

Dosage Forms & Route of Administration
2.5-mg oral tablets; 5-, 50-mg vials; IV and IM

Mechanism of Action
Antimetabolite (folic acid antagonist): the drug binds reversibly to dihydrofolate reductase, preventing the conversion of dihydrofolate to tetrahydrofolate, which is necessary for purine/pyrimidine biosynthesis, and DNA synthesis.

Indications, Dosage & Duration of Treatment
Acute lymphoblastic leukemia: induction — 3.3 mg/M^2 orally in combination with prednisone 60 mg/M^2 daily; maintenance — 30 mg/M^2 twice weekly orally or IM, or 2.5 mg/kg IV every 14 days. Multiple drug therapy is used frequently.

Choriocarcinoma (females): 15–30 mg/day orally or IM for 5 days, repeated approximately every 2 to 3 weeks.

Solid tumors of head, neck, breast, bone, testes, and pelvis: 50–60 mg/M^2 weekly.

Meningeal leukemia: 0.2–0.5 mg/kg (maximum 12 mg) intrathecally every 2–5 days until cell count of cerebral spinal fluid returns to normal.

Rate of Administration
The drug may be given by IV push or by continuous infusion.

Absorption, Metabolism, Excretion
Oral absorption is rapid. Peak serum levels are obtained within one-half to 2 hours following IV or IM administration and within 1–4 hours with oral administration. Fifty percent is bound to plasma proteins. Metabolism is insignificant. Fifty to 90% is excreted unchanged in the urine within 24 hours. The drug appears to sequester in effusions. Significant CSF levels occur only with high dose, systemic, or intrathecal regimens. Drugs interfering with tubular secre-

tions, (e.g., penicillin, probenecid, cephalothin, sulfonamides) delay renal clearance.

Onset, Duration of Action, $T_{1/2}$
$T_{1/2}$ = 2–4 hours (oral and IM). Effect is proportional to tissue levels and duration.

Side Effects, Toxicity
Nausea, vomiting, abdominal distress, rash, anorexia, diarrhea, gastrointestinal ulceration, alopecia, bone marrow depression, megaloblastic anemia, stomatitis, vasculitis, pulmonary fibrosis, severe but self-limiting respiratory illness (with fever, cough, infiltrate, eosinophilia, and pleuritic pain), hepatotoxicity (both reversible enzyme elevations and cirrhosis), dermatologic complications (perifolliculitis, pigmentation, and rash), renal tubular necrosis, hyperuricemia, amenorrhea, sterility, paresthesia, decreased deep tendon reflexes, and depression. Arachnoiditis, encephalitis, and paraplegia may occur with itrathecal administration.

Contraindications
Severe renal or hepatic disease and preexisting bone marrow depression.

Clinically Significant Drug Interactions
Displacement from serum binding sites by salicylates, sulfonamides, phenytoin, tetracycline, chloramphenicol, and para-aminobenzoic acid. Ethanol may enhance liver toxicity. Vinca alkaloids increase the cellular uptake of the drug while penicillin, kanamycin, corticosteroids, hydroxyurea, bleomycin, and L-asparaginase decrease cellular uptake.

Notes
Oral administration is often preferred, since absorption is rapid and effective serum levels are obtained. Concurrent administration of allopurinol may prevent acute episodes of hyperuricemia but may also affect the antitumor capacity of the drug.

The drug slowly enters the systemic circulation after intrathecal administration and causes delayed myelosuppression. High-dose regimen with leucovorin "rescue" remains experimental.

In cases of methotrexate overdose or high-dose regimens, calcium leucovorin (citrovorum factor, folinic acid), a potent folic acid antagonist) should be administered as soon as possible. This bypasses the enzyme block by supplying depleted end products (i.e., reduced folate, thymidine, purines).

Forced diuresis and urinary alkalinization reduce the renal precipitation that occurs in high-dose regimens of the drug.

Avoid the use of live-virus vaccines in patients on methotrexate therapy.

Methotrexate levels should be monitored in all patients on high-dose regimens.

References

Anderson, L. L.; Collins, G. J.; Ojima, Y.; and Sullivan, R. D. A study of the distribution of methotrexate in human tissues and tumors. *Cancer Res.* 30:1344–48, 1970.

Bertino, J. R., and Johns, D. G. Folate antagonists. *Annu. Rev. Med.* 18:27–34, 1967.

Bleyer, W. A. Methotrexate — clinical pharmacology, current status and therapeutic guidelines. *Cancer Treat. Rev.* 4:87–101, 1977.

Capizzi, R. L.; De Conti, R. C.; Marsh, J. C.; and Bertino, J. R. Methotrexate therapy of head and neck cancer: improvement in therapeutic index by the use of leucovorin "rescue." *Cancer Res.* 30:1782–88, 1970.

Condit, P. T.; Chanes, R. E.; and Joel, W. Renal toxicity of methotrexate. *Cancer* 23:126–31, 1969.

Henderson, E. S.; Adamson, R. H.; and Oliverio, V. T. The metabolic fate of tritiated methotrexate. II. Absorption and excretion in man. *Cancer Res.* 25:1018–24, 1965.

Lane, M.; Moore, J. E., III; Levin, H.; and Smith, F. E. Methotrexate therapy for squamous cell carcinomas of the head and neck. *J. A. M. A.* 204:561–64, 1968.

Roenigk, H. H., Jr.; Bergfeld, W. F.; St. Jacques, R.; Owens, F. J.; and Hawk, W. A. Hepatotoxicity of methotrexate in the treatment of psoriasis. *Arch. Dermatol.* 103:250–61, 1971.

Sostman, H. D.; Matthay, R. A.; Putman, C. E.; and Smith, G. J. W. Methotrexate-induced pneumonitis. *Medicine* 55:317–88, 1976.

Stoller, R. G.; Hande, K. R.; Jacobs, S. A.; Rosenberg, S. A.; and Chabner, B. A. Use of plasma pharmacokinetics to predict and prevent methotrexate toxicity. *N. Engl. J. Med.* 297:630–34, 1977.

MITHRAMYCIN

Trade Name
Mithracin®

Classification Category
Natural Product (Antibiotic)

Dosage Forms & Route of Administration
2.5-mg vials; IV infusion

Mechanism of Action
The drug inhibits DNA-directed synthesis of RNA by directly complexing with DNA.

Indications, Dosage & Duration of Treatment
Embryonal cell carcinoma of the testes: 25–30 μg/kg by IV infusion daily or on alternate days for 8–10 doses or until toxicity develops.

Rate of Administration
IV: infusion over 4–6 hours in 1 liter of 5% Dextrose Injection, U.S.P.

Absorption, Metabolism, Excretion
The CSF levels are equivalent to the blood levels at 4–6 hours. Twenty-five percent of the drug is excreted in the urine in 2 hours.

Onset, Duration of Action, $T_{1/2}$

Side Effects, Toxicity
Anorexia; nausea and vomiting; diarrhea; stomatitis; bone marrow depression; hepatic damage with decreased production of factors II, V, VII, and X; vascular damage; thrombocytopenia; hemorrhagic diathesis with hypocalcemia; renal failure; facial flushing; fever; irritability; fibrinolysis and vascular platelet dysfunction; lethargy; and depression.

Contraindications
Liver or kidney dysfunction, coagulation disorders, or thrombocytopenia.

Clinically Significant Drug Interactions

Notes

The drug should be discontinued with signs of vasculitis (e.g., a flush or conjunctivitis); an elevation in BUN, LDH, or prothrombin time; or depression of platelet count.

The drug has been successful in a single 15–25μg/kg IV injection (repeated every 2–4 days as needed) for the treatment of severe hypercalcemia in association with malignancy even when the tumor is resistant to the cytotoxicity of the drug. Calcium reduction is probably due to direct suppression of osteoclasts, although it may also block parathormone production.

Liver, kidney, and bone marrow toxicity can occur separately or simultaneously.

Antiemetic drugs may be useful in preventing nausea and vomiting.

Store in refrigerator. Reconstitute with 4.9 ml Sterile Water for Injection, U.S.P. (pH = 7.0). The drug is unstable in acid pH. Use immediately after mixing.

Rapid IV infusion has been associated with a greater incidence and severity of gastrointestinal side effects. Avoid extravasation.

References

Brown, J. H., and Kennedy, B. J. Mithramycin in the treatment of disseminated testicular neoplasms. *N. Engl. J. Med.* 272:111–18, 1965.

Kennedy, B. J. Mithramycin therapy in advanced testicular neoplasms. *Cancer* 26:755–66, 1970.

Kofman, S., and Eisenstein, R. Mithramycin in the treatment of disseminated cancer. *Cancer Chemother. Rep.* 32:77–96, 1963.

Perlia, C. P.; Gubisch, N. H.; Wolter, J.; Edelberg, D.; Dederick, M. M.; and Taylor, S. G. III. Mithramycin treatment of hypercalcemia. *Cancer* 25:389–94, 1970.

Ream, N. W.; Perlia, C. P.; Wolter, J.; and Taylor, S. G. Mithramycin therapy in disseminated germinal testicular cancer. *J. A. M. A.* 204:1030–36, 1968.

MITOMYCIN C

Trade Name
Mutamycin®

Classification Category
Natural Product (Antibiotic)

Dosage Forms & Route of Administration
5-mg vial; IV injection

Mechanism of Action
After activation by intracellular reductases, the drug functions as an alkylating agent, cross-linking with DNA. The guanine and cytosine content correlates with the degree of mitomycin-induced cross-linking. At high concentrations of the drug, cellular RNA and protein synthesis is also suppressed.

Indications, Dosage & Duration of Treatment
Disseminated adenocarcinoma of the stomach or pancreas: 20 mg/M^2 IV or 2 mg/M^2 IV for 5 days with a 2-day rest period, followed by 2 mg/M^2 for 5 days IV for a total dose of 20 mg/M^2 over 12 days. Both regimens are repeated at 6- to 8-week intervals. The drug is not recommended as single-agent primary therapy. The drug is also active in head, neck, and breast cancer.

Rate of Administration
Rapid IV injection or infusion over 30 minutes.

Absorption, Metabolism, Excretion
The drug is rapidly cleared from the serum after IV administration. The rate of clearance is determined by metabolism in the liver, but metabolism occurs in other tissues as well. Approximately 20% of a dose is excreted unchanged in the urine. Since metabolic pathways are saturated at relatively low doses, the percentage of a dose excreted in the urine increases with increasing dose.

Onset, Duration of Action, $T_{1/2}$
Following a 30-mg bolus injection, the serum concentration is reduced by 50% in 17 minutes. After injection of 30 mg, 20 mg, or 10 mg IV, the maximal serum concentrations are approximately 2.4 μg/ml, 1.7 μg/ml, and 0.52 μg/ml, respectively.

Side Effects, Toxicity
Leukopenia, thrombocytopenia, cellulitis at injection site, stomatitis, alopecia, renal impairment (glomerular sclerosis), fever, anorexia, nausea, vomiting, headache, blurred vision, confusion, drowsiness, syncope, fatigue, edema, thrombophlebitis, hematemesis, and diarrhea.

Contraindications
Previously demonstrated hypersensitivity or idiosyncratic reaction, thrombocytopenia, and coagulation disorders or increased bleeding tendency due to other causes.

Clinically Significant Drug Interactions

Notes
Care should be taken to avoid extravasation of the compound. If extravasation occurs, cellulitis, ulceration, and sloughing may result.

Reconstitute with 10 ml of Sterile Water for Injection, U.S.P. Dilute in 50–100 ml 5% Dextrose Injection, U.S.P., for IV infusion.

Protect from light to avoid decomposition. Administer as soon as possible after reconstitution.

The drug is not cross-resistant with other alkylating agents.

References

Manheimer, L. H., and Vital, J. Mitomycin C in the therapy of far-advanced malignant tumors. *Cancer* 19:207–12, 1966.

Moertel, C. G.; Reitemeier, R. J.; and Hahn, R. G. Mitomycin C therapy in advanced gastrointestinal cancer. *J. A. M. A.* 204:1045–48, 1968.

Slack, N., and Rimm, A. A. Effects of mitomycin C (NSC-26980) in 346 patients with advanced cancer. *Cancer Chemother. Rep.* 52:675, 1968.

Watne, A. L.; Moore, D.; and Gorgun, B. Solid tumor chemotherapy with mitomycin C. *Arch. Surg.* 93:174–78, 1967.

Whittington, R. M., and Close, H. P. Clinical experience with mitomycin C (NSC-26980). *Cancer Chemother. Rep.* 54:195, 1970.

PREDNISONE

Trade Name
Varies

Classification Category
Hormone (Adrenocorticosteroid)

Dosage Forms & Route of Administration
5-, 10-, 20-mg oral tablets (various others)

Mechanism of Action
Lympholytic effect and suppression of mitosis in lymphocytes.

Indications, Dosage & Duration of Treatment
Acute and chronic lymphocytic leukemia, Hodgkin's disease and other lymphomas, myeloma, and carcinoma of the breast: in combination therapy use 40–100 mg/M^2 (see Protocols section).

Rate of Administration

Absorption, Metabolism, Excretion
Gastrointestinal absorption is rapid. Conjugation occurs primarily in the liver and to some extent in the kidney. The drug is rapidly eliminated by glomerular filtration and tubular secretion. Fifty percent of a single dose is excreted in 1–3 hours.

Onset, Duration of Action, $T_{1/2}$

Side Effects, Toxicity
Epigastric distress, weight gain, truncal obesity, striae, skin fragility, "moon face," peptic ulcers, osteoporosis, enhanced risk of infection, impaired glucose tolerance, hypertension, myopathy, and mental distrubances.

Contraindications
Contraindicated in patients with peptic ulcer, psychosis, acute glomerular nephritis, herpes simplex of the eye, exanthematous diseases, Cushing's syndrome, infections not controlled by antibiotics, and myasthenia gravis.

Clinically Significant Drug Interactions
Amphotericin B, oral anticoagulants, antidiabetic agents, barbiturates, chlorthalidone, phenytoin, estrogens, ethacrynic acid, furosemide, indomethacin, salicylates, and thiazide diuretics.

Notes
Consider prophylaxis of tuberculosis in patients with a history of TB or exposure to TB or with lymphoma. Use antacids for gastric distress.

Corticosteroids may be useful adjuncts to the management of hypercalcemia.

References

Ezdinli, E. Z.; Stutzman, L.; Aungst, C. W.; and Firat, D. Corticosteroid therapy for lymphomas and chronic lymphocytic leukemia. *Cancer* 23:900–909, 1969.

Hall, T. C.; Choi, O. S.; Abadi, A.; and Krant, M. J. High dose corticoid therapy in Hodgkin's disease and other lymphomas. *Ann. Intern. Med.* 66:1144–53, 1967.

Manheimer, L. H. Hypercalcemia of breast cancer: management with corticosteroids. *Cancer* 18:679, 1965.

PROCARBAZINE

Trade Name
Matulane®

Classification Category
Miscellaneous Agent (Methylhydrazine Derivative)

Dosage Forms & Route of Administration
50-mg oral capsules

Mechanism of Action
The mechanism of action is not firmly established. Multiple sites of action have been postulated, including alkylation, oxidation of nucleic acids, and inhibition of transmethylation.

Indications, Dosage & Duration of Treatment
Hodgkin's disease: 100–200 mg/day (see Protocols section). Also active in glioblastoma multiforme, non-Hodgkin's lymphoma, and bronchogenic carcinoma.

Rate of Administration

Absorption, Metabolism, Excretion
Oral absorption is adequate and the drug is rapidly metabolized by the liver. Twenty-five to 75% of a dose is excreted in the urine within 24 hours. Less than 5% is excreted unchanged in the urine. The drug readily enters the CSF.

Onset, Duration of Action, $T_{1/2}$
Biological $T_{1/2}$ in plasma and CSF is approximately 1 hour.

Side Effects, Toxicity
Nervous system toxicity, such as confusion, depression, irritability, seizures, nystagmus, ataxia, and peripheral neuropathy with paresthesias (more common in elderly; related to amine oxidase inhibition); skin eruptions; mild hemolysis; orthostatic hypotension; myalgias; and arthralgias. Fifty to 70% of patients experience nausea and vomiting, leukopenia, and thrombocytopenia.

Contraindications
Known hypersensitivity to the drug, inadequate bone marrow reserve.

Clinically Significant Drug Interactions
Monoamine oxidase inhibitors, sympathomimetic amines, alcohol, local anesthetics, CNS depressants, tricyclic antidepressants, phenothiazines, and foods with high tyramine content.

Notes
It is essential that a complete blood count (with differential, reticulocyte, and platelet counts), blood chemistries, and urinalysis be done prior to therapy and at frequent intervals thereafter.

Temporary discontinuance of drug therapy is usually effective in controlling toxicity.

The use of antiemetics should be considered; however, phenothiazine antiemetics should be avoided due to CNS depression.

References

Raaflaub, J., and Schwartz, D. E. The metabolism of a cytostatic active methylhydrazine derivative (Matulane). *Experientia* 21:44–45, 1965.

Samuels, M. L.; Leary, W. V.; and Howe, C. D. Procarbazine (NSC-77213) in the treatment of advanced bronchogenic carcinoma. *Cancer Chemother. Rep.* 53:135–45, 1969.

Spivack, S. D. Procarbazine. *Ann. Intern. Med.* 81:795–800, 1974.

Stolinsky, D. L., *et al.* Procarbazine HCl in Hodgkin's disease, reticular cell sarcoma and lymphosarcoma. *Proc. Am. Assoc. Cancer Res.* 10:88, 1969.

SEMUSTINE (MeCCNU)

Trade Name
(Investigational NSC-95441)

Classification Category
Alkylating Agent (Nitrosourea)

Dosage Forms & Route of Administration
10-, 50-, 100-mg oral capsules

Mechanism of Action
The biochemical effects have not yet been worked out as they have for BCNU, although the mechanism of action may be similar to that of BCNU. The following actions have been attributed to BCNU:

a. Alkylation by formation of diazohydroxide and/or 2-chlorethylamine.

b. Selective interference with the utilization of histidine in 1-carbon metabolism in *de novo* purine synthesis through inhibition of formimino-transferase or cyclodeaminase.

c. Increased NADase activity and decrease in concentration of NAD^+ in tumor cells.

d. Decreased DNA nucleotidyl-transferase activity.

Indications, Dosage & Duration of Treatment
Adenocarcinoma of the gastrointestinal tract and advanced non-Hodgkin's lymphoma: 150mg/M^2 PO every 6 weeks. Treatment is discontinued upon first signs of progressive disease. Possibly effective in multiple myeloma and glioblastoma multiforme.

Rate of Administration

Absorption, Metabolism, Excretion
The drug is rapidly absorbed after oral administration. Evidence indicates that the parent compound is probably not the active agent, since the parent compound is rapidly metabolized. The metabolite

or metabolites are as yet unknown. Urinary excretion of the metabolite is virtually complete in 48–72 hours.

Onset, Duration of Action, $T_{1/2}$
Significant plasma levels having a half-life of 36–72 hours, can be seen as early as 10 minutes after administration.

Side Effects, Toxicity
Cumulative thromocytopenia and leukopenia, anemia, anorexia, nausea, vomiting, alopecia, and mucositis.

Contraindications

Clinically Significant Drug Interactions

Notes
Use antiemetics for nausea and vomiting. Store in refrigerator. Take with fluids on an empty stomach. Monitor renal, hepatic, and bone marrow functions.

References

Sponzo, R. W.; DeVita, V. T.; and Oliveria, V. T. Physiologic disposition of 1-(2-chloroethyl)-3-cyclohexyl-1-nitrosourea (CCNU) and 1-(2-chloroethyl)-3-(4-methyl cyclohexyl)-1-nitrosourea (MeCCNU) in man. *Cancer* 31:1154–59, 1973.

Wasserman, T. H.; Slavik, M.; and Carter, S. K. Methyl-CCNU in clinical cancer therapy. *Cancer Treat. Rev.* 1:251–69, 1974.

Wasserman, T. H.; Slavik, M.; and Carter, S. K. Clinical comparison of the nitrosoureas. *Cancer* 36:1258–68, 1975.

STREPTOZOTOCIN

Trade Name
(Investigational NSC-85998)

Classification Category
Alkylating Agent (Nitrosourea)

Dosage Forms & Route of Administration
1.0-gm lyophilized vials; IV

Mechanism of Action
Direct inhibition of DNA, RNA, and protein synthesis. The drug also inhibits the progress of cells into mitosis from G_2 of the cell cycle. The glucosamine moiety permits selective transport into pancreatic beta cells.

Indications, Dosage & Duration of Treatment
Metastatic islet-cell carcinoma of the pancreas and metastatic carcinoid: 500 mg/M^2 IV bolus daily for 5 days, to be repeated every 4 to 6 weeks, or 1 gm/M^2/week for 4 weeks. The drug is also active as second-line therapy in Hodgkin's disease.

Rate of Administration
IV infusion over 15–30 minutes.

Absorption, Metabolism, Excretion
Oral absorption is poor. No unchanged drug is detectable 3 hours after administration. Drug excretion occurs primarily in the urine. At 4 hours, less than 10% of the drug is recovered unchanged in the urine; at 24 hours this rises to only 11%. Less than 1% of the drug is recovered in the feces. One hour after administration CSF levels of the drug are approximately one-third of the plasma levels of the drug. CSF and plasma levels become equal at 2 hours.

Onset, Duration of Action, $T_{1/2}$
Radioactively labeled streptozotocin demonstrates a triphasic fall in plasma radioactivity and first-order kinetics. The initial phase $T_{1/2} = 6$ minutes; the second phase $T_{1/2} = 3.5$ hours; and the third phase $T_{1/2} \geq 40$ hours.

Side Effects, Toxicity

Nausea, vomiting, diarrhea, reversible liver function abnormalities, and myelosuppression (to varying degrees). The most serious toxic effects are renal, ranging from minimal proteinuria and azotemia to a complete Fanconi's syndrome with hypophosphatemia and renal tubular acidosis. Renal effects are usually transient, but may become life-threatening or fatal if treatment is continued after renal toxicity becomes manifest. Toxicity is not predictable on the basis of pretreatment renal function. Ataxia has been reported and chills, transient insulinism, and drug-induced diabetes have been observed.

Contraindications

Significant renal dysfunction.

Clinically Significant Drug Interactions

Notes

Reconstitute with 9.3 ml Sterile Water for Injection, U.S.P., or Sodium Chloride for Injection, U.S.P. Intact vials should be stored under refrigeration. Reconstituted solutions are chemically stable for at least 48 hours at room temperature. Brown discoloration occurs with decomposition.

The absence of preservatives precludes dispensing in multi-dose vials.

Renal function must be monitored periodically.

Drug therapy should not be initiated in patients with a creatinine clearance of less than 60 ml/minute.

The diabetogenic effect can be prevnted by prior treatment with nicotinamide.

In the treatment of any functioning islet-cell tumor, transient significant clinical exacerbation of symptoms may occur as a consequence of the release of insulin. The dose should be decreased 50% of the standard dose, then escalated to 100% on the second course if severe symptoms do not occur.

Consider the use of antiemetics.

References

Broder, L. E., and Carter, S. K. Pancreatic islet cell carcinoma II. Results of therapy with streptozotocin in 52 patients. *Ann. Intern. Med.* 79:108–18, 1973.

Moertel, C. G.; Reitemeier, R. J.; Schutt, A. J.; and Hahn, R. G. Phase II study of streptozotocin (NSC-85998) in the treatment of advanced gastrointestinal cancer. *Cancer Chemother. Rep.* 55:303–7, 1971.

National Cancer Institute. *Guideline for the clinical use of streptozotocin (NSC-85998).* Bethesda, Maryland, 1976.

Rakieten, P.S.; Rakeiten, M. L.; and Nadkarni, M. V. Studies of the diabetogenic action of streptozotocin. *Cancer Chemother. Rep.* 29:91–98, 1962.

Sadoff, L. Nephrotoxicity of streptozotocin (NSC-85998). *Cancer Chemother. Rep.* 54:457, 1970.

Schein, P. S.; Cooney, D. A.; and Vernon, M. L. The use of nicotinamide to modify the toxicity of streptozotocin diabetes without loss of antitumor activity. *Cancer Res.* 27:2324–32, 1967.

TAMOXIFEN CITRATE

Trade Name
Nolvadex®

Classification Category
Hormone (Antiestrogen)

Dosage Forms & Route of Administration
10-mg oral tablets

Mechanism of Action
Inhibits estrogen binding in breast cancer cells that contain estrogen receptors.

Indications, Dosage & Duration of Treatment
Palliative treatment of advanced breast cancer in postmenopausal women: 10–20 mg twice daily.

Rate of Administration

Absorption, Metabolism, Excretion
Peak levels are attained in 4–7 hours after dosing, with only 20–30% of the drug present as tamoxifen. The drug is slowly excreted in the feces, and only a small amount appears in the urine. The drug is excreted mainly as conjugates, with unchanged drug and hydroxylated metabolites accounting for 30% of the total.

Onset, Duration of Action, $T_{1/2}$
The initial half-life is 7–14 hours; secondary peaks occur 4 or more days later. The prolongation of blood levels and fecal excretion is believed to be due to enterohepatic circulation.

Side Effects, Toxicity
Hot flashes, nausea, vomiting, vaginal bleeding, vaginal discharge, menstrual irregularities, skin rash, hypercalcemia, peripheral edema, distaste for food, pruritis vulvae, depression, dizziness, lightheadedness, and headache.

Contraindications
There are no known contraindications.

Clinically Significant Drug Interactions

Increased bone and tumor pain and local disease flare have occurred. These may be associated with a good tumor response. The drug may cause increased bone and tumor pain requiring additional analgesics. Patients with soft-tissue disease may experience sudden increases in size of preexisting lesions. This may be associated with marked erythema within and surrounding the lesions and/or the development of new lesions. When this occurs, the bone pain or disease flare is seen shortly after starting tamoxifen and generally subsides rapidly. The response rates approach 60–70% in patients with estrogen receptors and in patients previously responding to hormonal manipulation.

References

Heel, R. C.; Brogden, R. N.; Speight, J. M., et al. Tamoxifen: a review of its pharmacologic properties and therapeutic use in the treatment of breast cancer. *Drugs* 16:1–24, 1978.

Kiang, D. T., and Kennedy, B. J. Tamoxifen (antiestrogen) therapy in advanced breast cancer. *Ann. Intern. Med.* 87:687–90, 1977.

Legha, S. S., and Carter, S. K. Antiestrogens in the treatment of breast cancer. *Cancer Treat. Rev.* 3:205–16, 1976.

Legha, S. S.; Davis, H. L.; and Muggia, F. M. Hormonal therapy of breast cancer: new approaches and concepts. *Ann. Intern. Med.* 88:69–77, 1978.

Lerner, J. H.; Band, P. R.; Israel, L.; and Leung, B. S. Phase II study of tamoxifen: report of 74 patients with Stage IV breast cancer. *Cancer Treat. Rep.* 60:1421–35, 1976.

McGuire, W. L. Current status of estrogen receptors in human breast cancer. *Cancer* 36:638–44, 1975.

McGuire, W. L.; Carbone, P. P.; and Vollner, E. P., eds. *Estrogen receptors in human breast cancer.* New York: Raven Press, 1975.

Stuart Pharmaceuticals. Clinical Drug Brochure. *Tamoxifen Citrate.* Wilmington, Delaware, 1978.

Ward, H. W. Anti-estrogen therapy for breast cancer: a trial of tamoxifen at two dose levels. *Brit. Med. J.* 1:13–14, 1973.

TESTOSTERONE SALTS
(Enanthate, Cypionate, Propionate)

Trade Name
Oreton®, Depo-Testosterone cypionate®, Delatestryl®, Ditate-DS®

Classification Category
Hormone (Androgen)

Dosage Forms & Route of Administration
10-mg buccal tablets; 50, 100, 200 mg/ml injections

Mechanism of Action
The mode of action is postulated to be a direct inhibitory effect on breast tumor tissue and secretion of pituitary gonadotropic hormones and prolactin, as well as an antiestrogenic effect on the tumor.

Indications, Dosage & Duration of Treatment
For palliation of breast cancer: 150–300 mg weekly, in 3 divided doses. Androgens should be continued for at least 2 months to achieve a satisfactory subjective response. Responders are usually continued on therapy until there is evidence of progressive disease.

Rate of Administration

Absorption, Metabolism, Excretion
The drug is distributed throughout most tissues, conjugated primarily in the liver and in the kidneys, and rapidly eliminated by glomerular filtration and tubular secretion.

Onset, Duration of Action, $T_{1/2}$

Side Effects, Toxicity
Occasional nausea and vomiting, occurring more frequently at higher doses. Hypercalcemia (10%), edema, and acceleration of the disease may occur and require early corrective measures.

Contraindications

Male breast or prostate carcinoma.

Clinically Significant Drug Interactions

Notes

Use with care in elderly patients with cardiac, liver, or renal disease; in patients with nephrotic syndrom (edema); and in immobilized patients, who are especially likely to develop hypercalcemia.

The 17 methyl-substituted androgens have been reported to cause cholestatic hepatitis.

The drug may cause a rise in hemoglobin and hematocrit.

The drug may maximize the leukopenic effect of alkylating agents and 5-FU.

References

Goldenberg, I. S.; Waters, N.; Ravdin, R. S.; Ansfield, F. J.; and Segaloff, A. Androgenic therapy for advanced breast cancer in women. *J. A. M. A.* 223:1267–68, 1973.

Segaloff, A. Hormone treatment of breast cancer. *J. A. M. A.* 234:1175–77, 1974.

Watson, G. W., and Tumer, R. L. Breast cancer: a new approach to therapy. *Brit. Med. J.* 1:1315, 1959.

6-THIOGUANINE

Trade Name

Thioguanine®, 6-TG

Classification Category

Antimetabolite (Purine Analogue)

Dosage Forms & Route of Administration

40-mg oral tablets

Mechanism of Action

The guanine analogue is converted *in vivo* into a nucleotide and is incorporated into DNA. It also inhibits purine-synthesizing enzymes by a feedback mechanism that depletes purine pools.

Indications, Dosage & Duration of Treatment

Acute leukemia and chronic myelocytic (granulocytic) leukemia (see Protocols section for dosages in combination therapy.)

Rate of Administration

Absorption, Metabolism, Excretion

Peak concentrations in the blood are reached 6–8 hours after oral administration, and approximately 40% of the dose is excreted in the urine within 24 hours. When thioguanine is administered to man, S-methylation occurs in the liver. 2-amino-6-methylthiopurine, rather than free thioguanine, appears in the urine. After 8 hours, inorganic sulfate becomes a major urinary metabolite.

Onset, Duration of Action, $T_{1/2}$

Side Effects, Toxicity

Nausea, vomiting, anorexia, diarrhea, stomatitis, rash, and bone marrow depression manifested by leukopenia, reticulocytopenia, anemia, and thrombocytopenia. Jaundice has been observed in some leukemia patients.

Contraindications
Impaired renal function (use cautiously), preexisting liver dysfunction, and preexisting bone marrow depression.

Clinically Significant Drug Interactions

Notes
Blood counts should be done at least once a week.

Small initial doses of thioguanine should be administered to patients with impaired renal function, in whom the drug may be excreted more slowly, resulting in a greater cumulative effect.

There is no known antagonist to thioguanine. When toxicity develops, prompt discontinuance of the drug is essential in order to avoid irreversible depression of the bone marrow.

Unlike mercaptopurine and azathioprine, thioguanine may be continued in the usual dosage when allopurinol is used concurrently.

Consider the use of antiemetics.

References

Ellis, D. B., and LePage, G. A. Biochemical studies of resistance to 6-thioguanine. *Cancer Res.* 23:436–43, 1963.

LePage, G. A. Incorporation of 6-thioguanine into nucleic acids. *Cancer Res.* 20:403–8, 1960.

LePage, G.A. Basic biochemical effects and mechanisms of action of 6-thioguanine. *Cancer Res.* 23:1202–6, 1963.

LePage, G. A., and Jones, M. Purinethols as feedback inhibitors of purine synthesis in ascites tumor cells. *Cancer Res.* 21:642–49, 1961.

Sartorelli, A. C., and LePage, G. A. Metabolic effects of 6-thioguanine II. *In vivo* and *in vitro* biosynthesis of nucleic acid purines. *Cancer Res.* 18:1329, 1958.

VINBLASTINE

Trade Name
Velban®

Classification Category
Natural Product (Vinca Alkaloid)

Dosage Forms & Route of Administration
10-mg vials; IV

Mechanism of Action
The drug appears to bind to or crystallize critical microtubular proteins of the mitotic spindle, thus preventing their proper polymerization and causing metaphase arrest (M-phase-specific). Interference with metabolic pathways of amino acids leading from glutamic acid to the citric acid cycle and to urea has been suggested.

Indications, Dosage & Duration of Treatment
Palliative treatment of lymphomas, including disseminated Hodgkin's disease, lymphocytic lymphoma, and reticulum-cell sarcoma (histiocytic lymphoma); advanced stages of mycosis fungoides; neuroblastoma; and Letterer-Siwe disease. The drug is also useful in combination therapy of testicular neoplasms. Dose as a single agent should be administered at weekly intervals, starting with an initial dose of 0.1 mg/kg and increasing in increments of 0.05 mg/kg until myelosuppression occurs.

Rate of Administration
IV push

Absorption, Metabolism, Excretion
Following IV administration, the drug is rapidly cleared from the blood and localized in body tissues. The drug is extensively metabolized, primarily in the liver, and slowly excreted in the urine and feces via the bile.

Onset, Duration of Action, $T_{1/2}$

Side Effects, Toxicity
Nausea, vomiting, anorexia, diarrhea, constipation, epigastric and abdominal pain, adynamic ileus, pharyngitis, stomatitis, vesiculation of the mouth, hemorrhagic enterocolitis, rectal bleeding, bleeding from old peptic ulcers, leukopenia, thrombocytopenia, numbness, paresthesis, peripheral neuritis, mental depression, loss of tendon reflexes, headache, and convulsions.

Contraindications
Leukopenia in the presence of bacterial infection.

Clinically Significant Drug Interactions

Notes
Avoid extravasation (may cause phlebitis and necrosis).

Consider the use of antiemetics.

References

Frei, E., III,; Franzino, A.; Shnider, B. I.; Costa, G. A.; Colsky, J.; Brindley, C. O.; Hosley, H.; Holland, J. F.; Gold, G. L.; and Jonsson, U. Clinical studies of vinblastine. *Cancer Chemother. Rep.* 12:125–29, 1961.

Sohier, W. D.; Wong, R. K. L.; and Aisenberg, A. C. Vinblastine in the treatment of advanced Hodgkin's disease. *Cancer* 22:467–72, 1968.

Wright, T. L., *et. al.* Vinblastine in neoplastic disease. *Cancer Chemother. Rep.* 23:169, 1963.

VINCRISTINE

Trade Name
Oncovin®

Classification Category
Natural Product (Vinca Alkaloid)

Dosage Forms & Route of Administration
1-, 5-mg vials; IV

Mechanism of Action
The drug appears to bind to or crystallize critical microtubular proteins of the mitotic spindle, thus preventing their proper polymerization and causing metaphase arrest.

Indications, Dosage & Duration of Treatment
Acute leukemia, Hodgkin's disease (combination therapy), lymphocytic lymphoma, histiocytic lymphoma, neuroblastoma, bronchogenic carcinoma, osteogenic sarcoma, and Ewing's sarcoma: 0.4–1 mg/M^2 weekly (do not exceed 2 mg).

Rate of Administration
Solution may be injected either directly into a vein or into the tubing of a running IV infusion over a period of about 1 minute.

Absorption, Metabolism, Excretion
Following IV administration, the drug is rapidly cleared from the blood, extensively metabolized in the liver, and excreted primarily via the bile. Less than 5% of a dose is excreted in the urine.

Onset, Duration of Action, $T_{1/2}$

Side Effects, Toxicity
Neurotoxicity (peripheral neuropathy, depressed deep tendon reflexes, paresthesias, weakness, cranial nerve defects, lethargy, and seizures), autonomic and central nervous system toxicity, alopecia, mild leukopenia, mild anemia, mild thrombocytopenia, nausea, vomiting, diarrhea, adynamic ileus (constipation and abdominal distention), stomatitis, and oral ulceration.

Contraindications

Reduce dosage in patients with obstructive jaundice or liver damage.

Clinically Significant Drug Interactions

Notes

Avoid extravasation (may cause phlebitis and necrosis). The drug is not cross-resistant with vinblastine.

References

Johnson, I. S.; Armstrong, J. G.; Gorman, M.; and Burnett, J. P. The vinca alkaloids: a new class of oncolytic agents. *Cancer Res.* 23:1390–1427, 1963.

Selawry, O. S.; Holland, J. F.; and Wolman, I. J. Effect of vincristine (NSC-67574) on malignant solid tumors in children. *Cancer Chemother. Rep.* 52:497, 1968.

Whitelaw, D. M., and Kim, H. S. Vincristine in the treatment of neoplastic disease. *Cancer Med. Assoc. J.* 90·1385–89, 1964.

Common Toxicities

Toxicity

Drug	Alopecia	Anaphylaxis or Fever	Carcinogenic	Cardiac	Dermatologic	Endocrine	Gastrointestinal	Hepatic	Myelosuppression	Neurologic	Pulmonary	Renal
Androgens		+				+		+				
Asparaginase		+				+	+	+ +		+ +		
Azacytidine		+			+		+ +					
Bleomycin		+ +			+ +		+				+ +	
Busulfan			+		+	+			+		+ +	
Carmustine (BCNU)			+		+		+	+	+			
Chlorambucil			+		+		+	+	+			
Cis-Platinum							+ +		+	+	+ +	
Corticosteroids					+	+	+/−					
Cyclophosphamide	+ +		+	+	+	+	+ +		+ +			+
Cytarabine		+				+	+	+	+			
Dacarbazine	+	+				+	+ +	+	+	+		

NOTE: Explanation of symbols: + = Toxic; + + = Moderately Toxic; + + + = Very Toxic; +/− = Variable

Toxicity

Drug	Alopecia	Anaphylaxis or Fever	Carcinogenic	Cardiac	Dermatologic	Endocrine	Gastrointestinal	Hepatic	Myelosuppression	Neurologic	Pulmonary	Renal
Dactinomycin	+ +				+		+ +		+ +			
Daunorubicin	+++	+		+ +			+ +		+ +			
Doxorubicin	+++	+		+ +	+		+ +		+ +			
Estrogens			+			+	+/−					
Fluorouracil	+				+		+ +		+ +	+		
Hexamethyl-melamine	+/−				+		+ +		+	+		
Hydroxyurea	+				+		+		+ +			+/−
Lomustine (CCNU)	+		+				+	+	+			
Mechlorethamine			+		+		+ +		+ +	+		
Melphalan			+ +				+		+			
Mercaptopurine							+	+ +	+			
Methotrexate	+				+		+ +		+ +	+	+	+
Mithramycin		+			+		+ +		+ +	+		

Toxicity

Drug	Fever	Anaphylaxis or Fever	Carcinogenic	Cardiac	Dermatologic	Endocrine	Gastrointestinal	Hepatic	Myelosuppression	Neurologic	Pulmonary	Renal
Mitomycin C	+				+		+ +		+		+	+
Mitotane (*o,p′*-DDD)	+				+	+	+ +			+ +		
Procarbazine		+	+ +		+	+	+ +		+ +	+ +		
Progesterone	+											
Semustine (MeCCNU)							+	+	+			+
Streptozotocin						+	+	+	+			+ +
Tamoxifen	+				+	+	+/−					
Thioguanine							+		+			+
Triethylenethiophosphoramide (Thiotepa®)		+					+ +		+ +			
Vinblastine							+		+ +	+		
Vincristine	+						+		+/−	+ +		

General References

American Society of Hospital Pharmacists. *American Hospital Formulary Service.* Washington, D. C., 1978.

Bender, R. A.; Zwelling, L. A.: Doroshow, J. H.; Locker, G. Y.; Hande, K. R.; Murinson, D. S.; Cohen, M.: Meyers, C. E.; Chabner, B. A. Antineoplastic drugs: clinical pharmacology and therapeutic use. *Drugs* 16:16–87, 1987.

Bodey, G. P., and Frei, E. III. Medical therapy of cancer. In *Harrison's: principles of internal medicine,* 7th ed., ed. M. M. Wintrobe, G. W. Thorn, R. D. Adams, E. Braunwald, K. J., Isselbacher, and R. G. Petersdorf, pp. 1736–99. New York: McGraw-Hill Book Company, 1977.

Calabresi, P., and Parks, R. E., Jr. Chemotherapy of neoplastic disease. In *The pharmacological basis of therapeutics,* 5th ed., ed. L. S. Goodman and A. Gilman, pp. 1248–1307. New York, The Macmillan Company, 1975.

Carter, S. K.; Bakowski, M. T.; and Hellman, K. *Chemotherapy of cancer.* New York: Wiley Medical, 1977.

Carter, S. K., and Slavik, M. Investigational drugs under study by the United States National Cancer Institute. *Cancer Treat. Rev.* 3:43–60, 1976.

Chabner, B. A., et. al. The Clinical Pharmacology of Antineoplastic Agents. *N. Engl. J. of Med.* 292: 1107–13, 1159-68, 1975.

Chabner, B. A.; Myers, C. E.; Oliverio, V. T. Clinical pharmacology of anticancer drugs. *Sem. Oncol.* 4: 165, 1977.

Clarysse, A., and Mathe, G. Malignant diseases. In *Drug treatment — principles and practice of clinical pharmacology and therapeutics,* ed. G. S. Avery, pp. 717–70. Acton, Mass.: Publishing Sciences Group, 1976.

Cline, M. J. *Major problems in internal medicine.* Cancer Chemotherapy, Vol. I. Philadelphia: W. B. Saunders Company, 1971.

Greenspan, E. M. *Clinical cancer chemotherapy.* New York: Raven Press, 1975.

Hansten, P. D. *Drug Interactions.* 3d ed. Philadelphia: Lea and Febiger, 1975.

Holland, J. F., and Frei, E., III. *Cancer Medicine.* Philadelphia: Lea and Febiger, 1975.

Marsh, J. C., and Mitchell, M. S. Chemotherapy of cancer: I. Overview of clinical pharmacology. II. Therapy of hematologic cancers. III. Therapy of solid tumors. *Drug Ther.* 4:87–114, 1974.

Oberfield, R. A., ed. Symposium on malignant disease. In *Medical clinics of North America,* vol 59, no. 2. Philadelphia: W. B. Saunders, 1975.

Owens, A. H. Predicting anti-cancer drug effects in man from animal studies. *J. Chronic Dis.* 15:223–28, 1962.

Pinkel, D. The use of body surface area as a criteria of drug dosage in cancer chemotherapy. *Cancer Res.* 18:853–56, 1958.

Silver, R. T.; Lauper, R. D.; and Jarowski, C. I. *A synopsis of cancer chemotherapy.* New York: Dun Donnelley Publishing Corp., 1977.

Skipper, H. E. Biochemical, biological, pharmacologic, toxicologic, kinetic, and clinical relationships. *Cancer* 21:600–610, 1968.

University of Texas System Cancer Center, M. D. Anderson Hospital and Tumor Institute. *Outlined guide for use of cancer chemotherapeutic agents.* Houston, 1975.

U. S. Department of Health, Education and Welfare, NIH, NCI, Division of Cancer Treatment. *Compilation of clinical protocol summaries.* 2nd ed. (DHEW publication no. (NIH) 78–1116.) Washington, D. C., 1977.

Warren, R. D.; Bender, R. A. Drug interactions with antineoplastic agents. *Cancer Treat. Rep.* 61:1231–41, 1977.

6

Newer Cancer Chemotherapeutic Drugs

1. Group A Drugs: limited to Division of Cancer Treatment — supported Phase I and early Phase II studies.

   α-TGdR (NSC-71851)
   Amino-thiadiazole (NSC-4728)
   AMSA (NSC-249992)
   Anguidine (NSC-141537)
   Bruceantin (NSC-165563)
   Chlorozotocin (NSC-178248)
   3-Deazauridine (NSC-126849)
   Dichloroallyl Lawsone (NSC-126771)
   Dichloromethotrexate (NSC-29630)
   Gallium Nitrate (NSC-15200)
   Hycanthone (NSC-142982)
   Maytansine (NSC-153858)
   Misonidazole (NSC-262047D) (Formerly Ro-07-0582)
   Neocarzinostatin (NSC-157365)
   Rubidazone (NSC-164011)

2. Group B Drugs: available for late Phase II (and beyond) studies by cooperative group members, Division of Cancer Treatment Contractors, and for certain drugs, cancer-center-affiliated investigators.

   a. Drugs available through the New Drug Studies mechanism:

Baker's Antifol (NSC-139105)
β-TGdR (NSC-71261)
Camptothecin (NSC-100880)
Cyclocytidine (NSC-145668)
Dianhydrogalactitol (NSC-132313)
Dibromodulcitol (NSC-104800)
Dibromomannitol (NSC-94100)
Elliott's B Solution (NSC-C-7) (Diluent)
ICRF-159 (NSC-129943)
Melphalan (I.V.) (NSC-8806)
Methyl-GAG (NSC-32946)
Streptonigrin (NSC-45383)
TMCA (NSC-36354)
Tubercidin (NSC-56408)
VM-26 (NSC-122819)
VP 16-213 (NSC-141540)
Yoshi 864 (NSC-102627)

b. Available only to Division of Cancer Treatment contractors and cooperative group studies:

Azaserine (NSC-742)
BCG-Connaught (NSC-B116341)
BCG-Pasteur (NSC-B116328)
BCG-Tice (NSC-B116327)
Calcium Leucovorin (NSC-3590)
C-Parvum (NSC-220537)
Cycloleucine (NSC-1026)
*DES (NSC-3070)
Erwinia Asparaginase (NSC-106977)
Estradiol Mustard (NSC-112259E)
*Fluoxymesterone (NSC-12165E)
Ftorafur (NSC-148958)
Isophosphamide (NSC-109724)
Levamisole (NSC-177023)
MER-BCG (NSC-143769)
6-Mercaptopurine (I.V.) (NSC-755)
Methotrexate (High Dose) (NSC-740)

Phenestrine (NSC-104469)
Piperazinedione (NSC-135758)
*Prednisolone (NSC-9151E)
*Prednisone (NSC-10023)
Procarbazine (I.V.) (NSC-77213)
Pyrozarurin (NSC-143095)
Rifamycin SV (NSC-133100)

* Special formulations.

3. Group C Drugs: Available to physicians who meet the following requirements:

   (1) A physician must be registered with the National Cancer Institute as an investigator.

   (2) Written request for the drug, indicating the disease to be treated, must be submitted.

   (3) The use of the drugs shall be limited to indications outlined in the guidelines that will be provided to the investigator.

   (4) All adverse reactions must be reported to the Investigational Drug Branch.

   Group C drugs with their approved indications are listed below:

Drug	*Approved Indication*
5-Azacytidine (NSC-102816)	Refractory acute myelogenous leukemia (AML)
Daunorubicin (NSC-82151)	AML and ALL
Streptozotocin (NSC-85998)	Islet-cell carcinoma of the pancreas, carcinoid
Semustine (MeCCNU) (NSC-95441)	Carcinoma of the colon and stomach, melanoma
Hexamethylmelamine (NSC-13875)	Ovarian carcinoma

Reference

Rubin, D. J., and Lewis, B. J., eds. Investigational drug distribution. *Division of Cancer Treatment Newsletter,* no. 4, pp. 1–3. United States Department of Health, Education and Welfare, Bethesda, Maryland, 1978.

7

Acronyms

(Examples: Past and Present)

Acronym	Protocol (Source of Acronym)[1]
ABVD (see Protocols section)	*Hodgkin's Disease.* Combines Doxorubicin (Adriamycin®), Bleomycin, Vinblastine, and Dacarbazine (DTIC®).
ACFUCY (J. Edmondson, p. 120)*	*Epithelial Ovarian Carcinoma.* Combines Actinomycin-D (Dactinomycin), 5-Fluorouracil, and Cyclophosphamide.
A-COPP (B. Hoogstraten, p. 248)*	*Hodgkin's Disease (children).* Combines Doxorubicin (Adriamycin®), Cyclophosphamide, Vincristine (Oncovin®), Procarbazine, and Prednisone.

[1]Protocol source may not reflect the original publication of the acronym.

**Compilation of Clinical Protocol Summaries.* 2d ed. Department of Health, Education and Welfare Publication No. (NIH) 78-1116, 1977. (All information marked with an asterisk in this chapter is from this source.)

BACON (B. Hoogstraten, p. 217)*	*Extensive Squamous-Cell Carcinoma of Lung.* Combines Bleomycin, Doxorubicin (Adriamycin®), Lomustine (CCNU), Vincristine (Oncovin®), and Nitrogen Mustard (Mechlorethamine).
BAVIP (L. Schelpper, p. 251)*	*Advanced Hodgkin's Disease.* Combines Bleomycin, Doxorubicin (Adriamycin®), Vinblastine, Dacarbazine (DTIC®), and Prednisone.
BCOP (J. R. Durant, p. 257)*	*Non-Hodgkin's Lymphoma.* Combines Carmustine (BCNU), Cyclophosphamide, Vincristine (Oncovin®), and Prednisone.
BCVP (P. Carbone, p. 256)*	*Non-Hodgkin's Lymphoma.* Combines Carmustine (BCNU), Cyclophosphamide, Vincristine, and Prednisone.
BCVPP (P. Carbone, p. 244)*	*Advanced Hodgkin's Disease.* Combines Carmustine (BCNU), Cyclophosphamide, Vinblastine, Procarbazine, and Prednisone.
BHD (B. Hoogstraten, p. 274)*	*Disseminated Malignant Melanoma.* Combines Carmustine (BCNU), Hydroxyurea, and Dacarbazine (DTIC®).
BHD-V (B. Hoogstraten, p. 274)*	*Disseminated Malignant Melanoma.* Combines Carmustine (BCNU), Hydroxyurea, Dacarbazine (DTIC®), and Vincristine.
CA-BOP (J. R. Bateman, p. 265)*	*Diffuse Lymphoma.* Combines Cyclophosphamide, Doxorubicin (Adriamycin®), Bleomycin, Vincristine (Oncovin®), and Prednisone.

CAD

(J. R. Durant, p. 175)*

Acute Myelogenous Leukemia. Combines Cytosine Arabinoside (Cytarabine) and Daunorubicin.

CAF

(B. Hoogstraten, p. 18)*

Advanced Breast Carcinoma. Combines Cyclophosphamide, Doxorubicin (Adriamycin ®), and 5-Fluorouracil.

CAP

(B. Hoogstraten, p. 193)*

Chronic Lymphocytic Leukemia. Combines Cyclophosphamide, Doxorubicin (Adriamycin®), and Prednisone.

CA-Ve

(Kaplan *et al. Cancer* 36:796–803, 1975)

Hodgkin's Disease (Resistant to MOPP). Combines Lomustine (CCNU), Doxorubicin (Adriamycin®), and Vinblastine.

CCM

(R. Vincent, p. 206)*

Oat-Cell Lung Carcinoma. Combines Cyclophosphamide, Lomustine (CCNU), and Methotrexate.

CHO

(B. Hoogstraten, p. 205)*

Oat-Cell Cancer of the Lung. Combines Cyclophosphamide, Hydroxydaunorubicin (Doxorubicin), and Vincristine (Oncovin®).

CHOP

(McKelvey *et al. Proc. Am. Soc. Clin. Oncol.* 15:184, 1974)

Non-Hodgkin's Lymphoma. Combines Cyclophosphamide, Hydroxydaunorubicin (Doxorubicin), Vincristine (Oncovin®), and Prednisone.

CHOR

(see Protocols section) (Livingston *et al. Ann. Intern. Med.* 88:194–199, 1978)

Small-Cell Bronchogenic Carcinoma of the Lung. Combines Cyclophosphamide, Hydroxydaunorubicin (Doxorubicin), Vincristine (Oncovin®), and Radiation therapy.

CHVP

(J. S. Abbatucci, p. 262)*

Non-Hodgkin's Lymphoma. Combines Cyclophosphamide, Hydroxydaunorubicin (Doxorubicin), VM-26 (Prodophyllotoxin derivative), and Prednisone.

CMF

(Bull *et al. Proc. Am. Ass. Clin. Oncol. 16:246, 1975)*

Metastatic Breast Carcinoma. Combines Cyclophosphamide, Methotrexate, and 5-Fluorouracil.

CMF(P)

(see Protocols section) (G. P. Canellos *et al. Ann. Intern. Med.* 84:389–92, 1976)

Metastatic Breast Carcinoma. Combines Cyclophosphamide, Methotrexate, 5-Fluorouracil, and Prednisone.

C-MOPP

(P. Carbone, p. 244)*

Hodgkin's Disease. Combines Cyclophosphamide, Nitrogen Mustard (Mechlorethamine), Vincristine (Oncovin®), Procarbazine, and Prednisone.

COAP

(B. Hoogstraten, p. 194)*

Chronic Myelogenous Leukemia. Combines Cyclophosphamide, Vincristine (Oncovin®), Ara-C (Cytarabine), and Prednisone.

COM

(P. Levy, p. 230)*

Undifferentiated Bronchogenic Carcinoma. Combines Cyclophosphamide, Vincristine (Oncovin®), and Semustine (MeCCNU).

COMB

(J. R. Bateman, p. 219)*

Lung Carcinoma. Combines Cyclophosphamide, Vincristine (Oncovin®), Semustine (MeCCNU), and Bleomycin.

COMF

(B. Hoogstraten, p. 205)*

Oat-Cell Carcinoma of the Lung. Combines Cyclophosphamide, Vincristine (Oncovin®), Methotrexate, and 5-Fluorouracil.

Cooper's Regimen

(R. G. Cooper. *Proc. Am. Assoc. Cancer Res.* 10:15, 1969)

Breast Cancer. Combines 5-Fluorouracil, Methotrexate, Vincristine (Oncovin®), Cyclophosphamide, and Prednisone.

COP

(Luce *et al. Cancer* 28: 306–17, 1971)

Non-Hodgkin's Lymphoma. Combines Cyclophosphamide, Vincristine (Oncovin®), and Prednisone.

COPP

(see Protocols section) (G. Mukherji *et al. Cancer* 28:886–93, 1971)

Lymphoma. Combines Cyclophosphamide, Vincristine (Oncovin®), Procarbazine, and Prednisone.

CP

(P. Carbone, p. 256)*

Non-Hodgkin's Lymphoma. Combines Cyclophosphamide and Prednisone.

CVA + BMP

(R. E. Wittes, p. 207)*

Oat-Cell Carcinoma of the Lung. Combines Cyclophosphamide, Vincristine, Doxorubicin (Adriamycin®), Carmustine (BCNU), Methotrexate, and Procarbazine.

CVP

(see Protocols section) (C. M. Bagley *et al. Ann. Intern. Med.* 76:227–34, 1972)

Non-Hodgkin's Lymphoma. Combines Cyclophosphamide, Vincristine, and Prednisone.

Cy-VA-DIC

(see Protocols section) (J. A. Gottlieb. *Cancer Chemother. Rep.* 58:265–70, 1974)

Sarcoma. Combines Cyclophosphamide, Vincristine, Doxorubicin (Adriamycin®), and Dacarbazine (DIC).

DCCMP

(A. Hoshino, p. 189)*

Acute Myelocytic, Monocytic, or Refractory Lymphocytic Leukemia. Combines Daunorubicin, Cyclocytidine, 6-Mercaptopurine, and Prednisone.

DCMP

(A. Hoshino, p. 189)*

Acute Myelocytic, Monocytic, or Refractory Lymphocytic Leukemia. Combines Daunorubicin, Cytosine Arabinoside (Cytarabine), 6-Mercaptopurine, and Prednisone.

DOAP

(B. Hoogstraten, p. 180)*

Acute Leukemia. Combines Daunorubicin, Vincristine '(Oncovin®), Ara-C (Cytarabine), and Prednisone.

DZAPO

(D. Hammond, p. 173)*

Acute Myelogenous Leukemia (children). Combines Daunorubicin, Azacytidine. Ara-C (Cytarabine), Prednisone, and Vincristine (Oncovin®).

FAC

(see Protocols section)
(J. R. Blumenschein *et al.* *Am. Soc. Clin. Oncol. Proc. Clin. Oncol.* 15:193,1974.

Metastatic Breast Carcinoma. Combines 5-Fluorouracil, Doxorubicin (Adriamycin®), and Cyclophosphamide.

FCP

(Ahmann *et al. Proc. Am. Ass. Cancer Res.* 15:100, 1974)

Breast Cancer. Combines 5-Fluorouracil, Cyclophosphamide, and Prednisone.

FUM

(J. U. Gutternamn, p. 26)*

Advanced Metastatic Breast Carcinoma. Combines 5-Fluorouracil and Methotrexate.

HOP

(McKelvey *et al. Proc. Am. Soc. Clin. Oncol.* 15:184, 1974)

Non-Hodgkin's Lymphoma. Combines Hydroxydaunorubicin (Doxorubicin), Vincristine (Oncovin®), and Prednisone.

LAPOCA

(M. H. Donaldson, p. 158)*

Marrow Relapse/Acute Leukemia (children). Combines L-Asparaginase, Prednisone, Vincristine (Oncovin®), Cytosine Arabinoside (Cytarabine), and Doxorubicin (Adriamycin®).

MACC

(see Protocols section)
(A. P. Chahinian et. *al.* *J. A. M. A.* 237:2392–96, 1977)

Non-Oat-Cell Carcinoma of the Lung. Combines Methotrexate, Doxorubicin (Adriamycin®), Cyclophosphamide, and Lomustine (CCNU).

M-BACOD

(A. T. Skarin, p. 261)*

Advanced Non-Hodgkin's Lymphoma. Combines Methotrexate/Citrovorum Factor, Bleomycin, Doxorubicin (Adriamycin®), Cyclophosphamide, Vincristine (Oncovin®), and Dexamethasone.

MOPP

(see Protocols section) (DeVita *et al. Ann. Intern. Med.* 73:881–95, 1970)

Advanced Hodgkin's Disease. Combines Nitrogen Mustard (Mechlorethamine), Vincristine (Oncovin®), Procarbazine, and Prednisone.

MVPP

(British variant of MOPP) (Nicholson *et al. Brit. Med. J.* 3:7–10, 1970)

Generalized Hodgkin's Disease. Combines Mustine Hydrochloride, Vincristine, Procarbazine, and Prednisone.

NAC

(B. Hoogstraten, p. 217)*

Extensive Squamous-Cell Carcinoma of the Lung. Combines Nitrogen Mustard (Mechlorethamine), Doxorubicin (Adriamycin®), and Lomustine (CCNU).

OAP

(B. Hoogstraten, p. 182)*

Adult Acute Leukemia. Combines Vincritine (Oncovin®), Ara-C (Cytarabine), and Prednisone.

OPAL

(B. Hoogstraten, p. 183)*

Adult Acute Leukemia. Combines Vincritine (Oncovin®), Prednisone, and L-Asparaginase.

OPP

(B. Hoogstraten, p. 335)*

Recurrent Brain Tumors (children). Combines Vincristine (Oncovin®), Procarbazine, and Prednisone.

PATCO

(D. Hammond, p. 172)*

Acute Myelocytic, Myelomonocytic, and Erythroleukemia (children). Combines Prednisone, Cytosine Arabinoside (Ara-C), 6-Thioguanine, Cyclophosphamide, and Vincristine (Oncovin®).

POMP

(Rodriguez *et al.* *Cancer* 32:69–75, 1973)

Adult Acute Leukemia. Combines Purinethol® (6-Mercaptopurine), Vincristine (Oncovin®), Methotrexate, and Prednisone.

Pulse VAC

(Wilbur *et al.* *Cancer* 36:765–69, 1975)

Sarcoma. Combines Vincristine, Actinomycin D (Dactinomycin), and Cyclophosphamide given simultaneously.

ROAP

(R. S. Benjamin, p. 188)*

Acute Leukemia. Combines Rubidazone, Vincristine (Oncovin®), Cytosine Arabinoside (Ara-C), and Prednisone.

TAD

(J. R. Durant, p. 175)*

Acute Myelogenous Leukemia. Combines 6-Thioguanine, Cytosine Arabinoside (Ara-C), and Daunorubicin.

VAC

(Wilbur *et al.* Cancer 36:765–69, 1975)

Sarcoma. Combines Vincristine, Actinomycin D (Dactinomycin), and Cyclophosphamide.

VAP

(B. Hoogstraten, p. 182)*

Acute Leukemia. Combines Vincristine, Doxorubicin (Adriamycin®), and Prednisone.

VAT-D

(P. Carbone, p. 174)*

Acute Nonlymphocytic Leukemia. Combines Vincristine, Cytosine Arabinoside (Ara-C), 6-Thioguanine, and Daunorubicin.

VAV — *Oat-Cell Lung Carcinoma.* Combines VP-16, Doxorubicin (Adriamycin®), and Vincristine.

(R. Vincent, p. 206)*

VBAP — *Multiple Myeloma.* Combines Vincristine, Carmustine (BCNU), Doxorubicin (Adriamycin®), and Prednisone.

(B. Hoogstraten, p. 138)*

VCAP — *Multiple Myeloma.* Combines Vincristine, Cyclophosphamide, Doxorubicin (Adriamycin®), and Prednisone.

(B. Hoogstraten p. 138)*

VCMP — *Multiple Myeloma.* Combines Vincristine, Cyclophosphamide, Melphalan, and Prednisone.

(B. Hoogstraten, p. 138)*

8

Protocols

(Examples)

"The continuing challenge in the experimental chemotherapy of cancer is the design of agents or measures which are selective for the cancer cell."* It is with this thought in mind that the protocols currently used in the treatment of different cancers were devised by the various research organizations throughout the country.

The following list is not meant to be a complete list of all the current protocols, but is only a sample of those most frequently encountered.

*G. C. Mueller, The G_1 conversion: a target for cancer chemotherapy. *Cancer Res.* 29:2394–97, 1969.

1. **ABVD** (Hodgkin's Disease)

   A Doxorubicin (Adriamycin®)
   25 mg/M² IV, days 1 and 14

   B Bleomycin
   10 mg/M² IV, days 1 and 14

   V Vinblastine
   6 mg/M² IV, days 1 and 14

   D Dacarbazine (DTIC®)
   150 mg/M², days 1–5

   Course to be repeated every 28 days.

Reference

Bonadonna, B.; Zucali, R.; Monfardini, S.; DeLena, M.; and Uslenghi, C. Combination chemotherapy of Hodgkin's disease with adriamycin, bleomycin, vinblastine, and imidazole carboxamide versus MOPP. *Cancer* 36:252–59, 1975.

2. **Ara-C + Adriamycin®** (Induction Remission of Acute Myelocytic Leukemia)

Ara-C	Cytosine Arabinoside (Cytarabine) 100 mg/M² IV, as a continuous 24-hour infusion for 7–10 days
Adriamycin®	(Doxorubicin) 30 mg/M² IV, days 1–3

Reference

Preisler, H.D.: Bjornsson, S.; and Henderson, E. S. Adriamycin®-cytosine arabinoside therapy for adult acute myelocytic leukemia. *Cancer Treat. Rep.* 61:89–92, 1977

3. **CHOR** (Small-Cell Bronchogenic Carcinoma of the Lung)

   C Cyclophosphamide
   750 mg/M², days 1 and 22

   H Hydroxydaunorubicin (Doxorubicin)
   50 mg/M², days 1 and 22

   O Vincristine (Oncovin®)
   1 mg (no modification for body surface area)

   R Radiation therapy to lung field and prophylactic whole-brain irradiation; begins on day 42

Reference

Livingstone, R. B.; Moore, T. N.; Heilbrun, L.; Bottomley, R.; Lehane, D.; Rivkin, S. E.; and Thigpen, T. Small cell carcinoma of the lung: combined chemotherapy and radiation. *Ann. Intern. Med.* 88:194–99, 1978.

4. **Cis-Platinum, Vinblastine, and Bleomycin** (Disseminated Testicular Cancer)

   Cis-Platinum (*Cis*-diamminedichloroplatinum)
   20 mg/M² as 15-minute infusion for 5 days every 3 weeks

   Vinblastine
   *0.2 mg/kg daily for 2 days every 3 weeks

   Bleomycin
   30 units on days 2, 9, and 16 of each platinum course, given with the platinum 6 hours after vinblastine, and then weekly for a total of 12 weeks.

*Vinblastine dose will be reduced 25% to patients who have had previous radiotherapy.

Reference

Einhorn, L. H., and Donohue, J. *Cis*-diamminedichloroplatinum, vinblastine, and bleomycin and combination chemotherapy in disseminated testicular cancer. *Ann. Intern, Med.* 87:293–98, 1977.

5. **CMF(P)** (Metastatic Breast Carcinoma)

   C Cyclophosphamide
   100 mg/M² PO, days 1–14

   M Methotrexate
   60 mg/M² IV, days 1 and 8

   F 5-Fluorouracil
   700 mg/M² IV, days 1 and 8

   P Prednisone
   40 mg/M² PO, days 1–14

   Course to be repeated every 28 days.

Reference

Canellos, G.P.; Gold, G. L.; and Schein, P. S. Combination chemotherapy for advanced breast cancer: response and effect on survival *Ann. Intern. Med.* 84:389–92, 1976.

6. **CMF-VP** (Modified Cooper's Regimen for Metastatic Breast Carcinoma)

   C Cyclophosphamide
   100 mg/M² PO, days 1–14

   M Methotrexate
   40 mg/M² IV, days 1 and 8

   F 5-Fluorouracil
   600 mg/M² IV, days 1 and 8

   V Vincristine
   1 mg/M² IV, days 1 and 8

P Prednisone
40 mg/M^2 PO, days 1–14

Reference

Cooper, R. G. Combination chemotherapy in hormone resistant breast cancer. *Proc. Am. Assoc. Cancer Res.* 10:15, 1969.

7. **COPP** (Lymphoma)

C Cyclophosphamide
450 mg/M^2 IV, days 1, 8, and 28

O Vincristine (Oncovin®)
1.4 mg/M^2 IV, days 1 and 8

P Procarbazine
100 mg/M^2 PO, days 1–10

P Prednisone
40 mg/M^2 PO, days 1–14

Reference

Mukherji, G.; Yogada, A.; Oettgen, H. F.; and Krakoff, I. H. Cyclic chemotherapy in lymphoma. *Cancer* 28:886–93, 1971.

8. **CVP** (Non-Hodgkin's Lymphoma)

C Cyclophosphamide
400 mg/M^2 PO, days 1–5 and day 21; or
450 mg/M^2 IV, days 1 and 8

V Vincristine
1.4 mg/M^2 IV, days 1 and 8

P Prednisone
100 mg/M^2 PO, days 1–5

Reference

Bagley, C. M., Jr.; DeVita, V. T., Jr.; Berard, C. W.; and Canellos, G. P. Advanced lymphosarcoma: intensive cyclical combination chemotherapy with cyclophosphamide, vincristine, and prednisone. *Ann. Intern. Med.* 76:227–34, 1972.

9. **Cy-VA-DIC** (Sarcoma)

Cy Cyclophosphamide
400-500 mg/M² IV, day 2

V Vincristine (Oncovin®)
1.5 mg/M² IV, days 1, 8, and 15

A Doxorubicin (Adriamycin®)
50 mg/M² IV, day 2

DIC Dacarbazine
250 mg/M² IV, days 1–5

Reference

Gottlieb, J. A. Combination chemotherapy for metastatic sarcoma. *Cancer Chemother. Rep.* 58:265–70, 1974.

10. **Doxorubicin and BCNU** (Multiple Myeloma)

Doxorubicin
30 mg/M² IV every 3–4 weeks

BCNU Carmustine
30 mg/M² IV every 3–4 weeks

Reference

Alberts, D. S.; Durie, B. G. M.; and Salmon, S. E. Doxorubicin/BCNU chemotherapy for multiple myeloma in relapse. *Lancet* 1:926–28, 1976.

11. **FAC** (Metastatic Breast Carcinoma)

F 5-Fluorouracil
500 mg/M² IV, days 1 and 8

A Doxorubicin (Adriamycin®)
50 mg/M² IV, day 1

C Cyclophosphamide
500 mg/M², day 1

Course to be repeated every 3 weeks.

Reference

Blumenschein, G. R.; Cardenas, J. O.; Freireich, E. J.; and Gottlieb, J. A. FAC chemotherapy for breast cancer. *Proc. Annual Soc. Clin. Oncol.* 15:193, 1974.

12. **5-FU, MeCCNU, and Vincristine** (Advanced Colorectal Carcinoma)

5-FU	5-Fluorouracil 100 mg/kg IV bolus, days 1–5 and then every 7 days beginning at day 14
MeCCNU	Semustine 100 mg/M² PO on day 1 and every 6 weeks thereafter
Vincristine	1.4 mg/M² IV every 3 weeks beginning on day 1 (maximum dose is 2 mg per injection)

References

Carter, S. K. Current protocol approaches in large bowel cancer. *Semin. Oncol.* 3:433–43, 1976.

Moertel, C. G.; Schutt, A. J.; Hahn, R. G.; and Reitemeier, R. J. Brief communication: therapy of advanced colorectal cancer with a combination of 5-fluorouracil, methyl-1-3-*cis*-(2-chloroethyl)-1-nitrosourea and vincristine. *J. Natl. Cancer Inst.* 54:69–71, 1975.

13. **MACC** (Non–Oat-Cell Carcinoma of the Lung)

M Methotrexate
40 mg/M^2, days 1 and 21

A Doxorubicin (Adriamycin®)
40 mg/M^2, days 1 and 21

C Cyclophosphamide
400 mg/M^2, days 1 and 21

C Lomustine (CCNU)
30 mg/M^2, days 1 and 21

Vincristine may be added to the above regimen at a dose of 2 mg administered 30 minutes prior to administration of the other drugs. The initial doses of methotrexate and Adriamycin® are reduced 25% when vincristine is added.

Reference

Chahinian, A. P.; Arnold, D. J.; Cohen, J. M.; Purpora, D. P.; Jaffney, I. S.; Teirstein, A. S.; Kirschner, P. A.; Holland, J. F. Chemotherapy for bronchogenic carcinoma. *J. A. M. A.* 237:2392–96, 1977.

14. **MOPP** (Advanced Hodgkin's Disease)

M Nitrogen Mustard (Mechlorethamine)
6 mg/M^2 IV, days 1 and 8

O Vincristine (Oncovin®)
1.4 mg/M^2 IV, days 1 and 8

P Procarbazine
50 mg PO, day 1; 100 mg PO, day 2; 100 mg/M^2 PO, days 3–10

P Prednisone
40 mg/M^2 PO, days 1–10

Reference

Frei, M.; Luce, J. K.; Gamble, J. F.; Coltman, C. A.; Constanzi, J. S.;

Talley, R. W.; Monto, R. W.; Wilson, H. E.; Hewlett, J. S.; Delaney, F. C.; and Gehan, E. A. Combination chemotherapy in advanced Hodgkin's disease. *Ann. Intern. Med.* 79:376–82, 1973.

9

Common Oncologic Problems

This section provides a brief review of problems and complications associated with cancer chemotherapy. The information is presented in abbreviated form and serves as a general overview and treatment outline for the practitioner. These recommendations should be followed only as an adjunct to current, medically accepted diagnostic and therapeutic procedures. Specific management approaches are more comprehensively described in general medical texts and recent literature.

ANEMIA

1) Blood Loss/Iron Deficiency Anemia

Blood loss/iron deficiency anemia may occur secondary to gastrointestinal or genitourinary malignancy or as a result of drug-induced mucosal ulceration (5-fluorouracil, methotrexate, acetylsalicylic acid). Treatment recommendations should be based both on the training and the experience of individual clinicians and on the facilities available at a given institution. Individual experience is often of more importance than any specific treatment approach.

Treatment

Give whole blood for active bleeding and packed red cells for chronic bleeding if hemoglobin falls below 8–10 gm%. Treat iron deficiency with 320 mg ferrous sulfate orally, four times daily or with iron dextran (Imferon®) by intravenous infusion in normal saline over one hour. A test dose of 0.25 ml should be given, monitoring for anaphylaxis.

2) Megaloblastic Anemia

Megaloblastic anemia may result from nutritional deficiencies of folate or vitamin B_{12}, gastrectomy, radiation therapy or malignancies such as lymphoma, leukemia, head and neck cancer, and liver metastases. Drug therapy with agents such as folate antagonists, alkylating agents, pyrimidine antagonists (6-mercaptopurine, 6-thioguanine), purine antagonist (5-fluorouracil) or ribonucleotide reductase inhibitors (cytarabine, hydroxyurea, procarbazine) may cause megaloblastic anemia.

Treatment

Specific nutritional deficiencies may respond to folic acid given in an oral dose of 1–3 mg daily or cyanocobalamin given intramuscularly in a dose of 1000 mcg daily for 14 days and followed by repetitions once monthly. Discontinue chemotherapy only if the condition becomes severe.

3) Myelophthisis (Leukoerythroblastosis)

Myelophthisis may result from carcinoma (breast, lung, thyroid, prostate), multiple myeloma, melanoma, lymphoma, leukemia, and myelofibrosis.

Treatment

The underlying malignancy should be treated with adequate doses of chemotherapeutic agents despite low blood counts.

4) Anemia of Chronic Disease

Anemia of chronic disease may be seen with malignancy, infection, or a number of chronic disease states.

Treatment

Treatment should correct the underlying condition. Refractory cases may respond to oxymethalone in oral doses of 60 mg/M^2 daily for 3–4 months.

5) Immune Hemolysis

Immune hemolysis may develop from drug therapy (antibiotics, cyclophosphamide, methyldopa, procarbazine) or malignancies (lymphoma, chronic lymphocytic leukemia, multiple myeloma, ovarian tumor).

Microangiopathic hemolysis may occur in a number of adenocarcinomas, e.g., breast, lung, pancreas, prostate, or lung.

Treatment

Treatment consists of removing the offending agent or treating the underlying malignancy. This condition may respond to prednisone in oral doses of 1 mg/kg per day, or may require splenectomy. Cyclophosphamide in daily oral doses of 50–100 mg/M^2 may be beneficial. Folate (1–3 mg daily) is useful for patients with associated megaloblastosis. Patients with severe anemia may require blood transfusions, but these should be avoided if at all possible.

6) **Hypersplenism**

Anemia due to splenic sequestration may occur in patients with splenomegaly due to lymphomas and various carcinomas.

Treatment

Treatment consists of treating the underlying malignancy. Splenectomy should be considered in refractory cases.

7) **Chemotherapy**

Chemotherapeutic agents commonly associated with anemia include *cis*-platinum and the nitrosoureas, and more rarely, other alkylating agents, anthrocyclines, antimetabolites, and the vinca alkaloids.

Treatment

Treatment involves withholding the offending agent and transfusing as required.

NOTE: Leukocyte-poor blood is preferred for patients with leukocyte antibodies and for those who will receive prolonged transfusion support or marrow transplant. Unless the patient is symptomatic, actively bleeding or infected, transfusions can be withheld until hemoglobin falls to 8gm/100 ml or below.

References

Cline, M. J., and Berlin, N. I. Studies of the anemia of multiple myeloma. *Am. J. Med.* 33:520–25, 1962.

Cline, M. J., and Berlin, N. I. Anemia in Hodgkin's disease. *Cancer* 16:526–32, 1963.

Hyman, G. A. Anemia in malignant neoplastic disease. *J. Chron. Dis.* 16:546–66, 1963.

Jones, S. E. Autoimmune disorders and malignant lymphoma. *Cancer* 31:1092–98, 1973.

Masouredis, S. P. Preservation and Clinical Use of Erythrocytes and Whole Blood. In *Hematology*. ed. W. J. Williams; E. Beutler; A. J. Erslev; and R. W. Rundles. New York: McGraw-Hill, 1977, p. 1530.

Miller, W. V.; Wilson, M. J.; and Kalb, H. J. Simple methods for production of HLA antigen poor red blood cells. *Transfusion* 13:189–93, 1973.

BLEEDING

1) Tumor Ulceration

Tumor invasion of blood vessels is a major cause of hemorrhage in patients with cancer.

Treatment

Treatment is directed at controlling the underlying malignancy and using local measures to control bleeding.

2) Thrombocytopenia

Thrombocytopenia is a major cause of hemorrhage in patients with cancer. It may result from myelosuppressive treatment, myelophthisic marrow, hypersplenism, intravascular coagulation or immune thrombocytopenia with lymphoma or chronic lymphocytic leukemia. Life threatening hemorrhage is unusual unless the platelet count falls below 20,000 per ml blood or unless additional coagulation defects are present.

Treatment

The routine use of platelet transfusions in severely thrombocytopenic patients has reduced fatal hemorrhage by over 50 percent. Platelet transfusions of 4–6 units/M^2 every 8 hours should be used for active bleeding. In acute thrombocytopenia without bleeding, platelet transfusions of 4–6 units/M^2 every 2 to 3 days should be considered when the platelet count falls below 20,000 per ml blood or below 30,000 in the presence of fever. The underlying malignancy must be treated if the bone marrow is involved. Splenectomy is often beneficial and should be considered in severe hypersplenism. Immune thrombocytopenia may respond to prednisone, 1 mg/kg per day orally, or may require splenectomy. Consider cyclophosphamide 50–100 mg/M^2 daily in refractory cases.

3) Platelet Function Abnormality

Platelet function abnormality may be seen in acute myelogenous leukemia, chronic lymphocytic leukemia or plasma cell dyscrasia such as multiple myeloma and macroglobulinemia.

Treatment

In conditions of platelet function abnormality with active bleeding, consider platelet transfusions of 4–6 units/M^2 every 8 hours.

4) Disseminated Intravascular Coagulopathy (DIC)

Disseminated Intravascular Coagulopathy is seen in patients with infection, acute leukemia (promyelocytic or monocytic), lymphoma (histiocytic), carcinomatosis (pancreas, prostate, lung), surgical complications, anaphylaxis, and transfusion reaction.

Treatment

Treat underlying malignancies. Use appropriate antibiotics for presumed sepsis. Consider heparin (10–20 units/kg per hour by continuous IV infusion), fresh frozen plasma, and platelet transfusion in severely affected refractory patients. Heparin prophylaxis in patients with promyelocytic leukemia may be effective.

5) Clotting Factor Deficiency

Bleeding may result from clotting factor deficiency as a result of disseminated intravascular coagulopathy (DIC), liver disease, drug therapy (6-mercaptopurine, methotrexate, L-asparaginase, androgenic agents), and circulating anticoagulants.

Treatment

Treatment includes the administration of fresh frozen plasma to control bleeding, vitamin K in patients with liver disease, and withdrawal of offending agents.

6) Primary Fibrinolysis

Primary fibrinolysis associated with pancreatic and prostatic carcinomas is rare and must be distinguished from secondary fibrinolysis.

Treatment

Primary fibrinolysis is treated with heparin 10- 20 units/kg per hour by continuous infusion and epsilon-aminocaproic acid 4 gm IV push followed by 1 gm per hour until bleeding is controlled. Limit the administration of epsilon-aminocaproic acid (Amicar®) to 30 gm per 24 hours.

7) **Paraproteinemia (IgG, IgM)**

The hyperviscosity syndrome, asociated with plasma cell dyscrasias, should be considered for patients with immunoglobin abnormalities.

Treatment

If symptoms are present or if serum viscosity is greater than three, plasmapheresis is used to treat paraproteinemia. Treatment should include chemotherapy for the underlying malignancy.

NOTE: Indications for transfusions depend upon the rate of bleeding. For rapid bleeding, transfuse with whole blood or packed red cells and plasma expanders to maintain stable vital signs and a hemoglobin of 10 gm%. For slow or occult bleeding, transfuse with packed red cells if hemoglobin is 8 gm% or less.

Menstruation during intensive therapy associated with thrombocytopenia may result in life-threatening hemorrage and may be managed prophylactically with conjugated estrogen (Premarin®), 5 mg daily by mouth.

References

Drapkin, R. L.; Gee, T. S.; Dowling, M. D.; et al. Prophylactic heparin therapy in acute promyelocytic leukemia. *Cancer* 41:2484–90, 1978.

Gaydos, L. ; Freireich, E. J.; and Mantel, N. Quantitative relation between platelet count and hemorrhage in patients with acute leukemia. *N. Eng. J. Med.* 266:905-9, 1962.

Gralnick, H. R., and Henderson, E. S. Acquired coagulation factor deficiencies in leukemia. *Cancer* 26:1097–2003, 1970.

Han, T.; Stutzman, L.; Cohen, E.; and Kim, U. Effect of platelet transfusion on hemorrhage in patients with acute leukemia. *Cancer* 19:1937–42, 1966.

Higby, D. J.; Cohen, E.; Holland, J.; et al. The prophylactic treatment of thrombocytopenic leukemic patients with platelets: a double blind study. *Transfusion* 14:440–46, 1974.

Lyman, G. H.; Bettigole, R.; Robson, E.; Ambrus, J. L.; and Urban, H. Fibrinogen kinetics in patients with neoplastic disease. *Cancer* 41:1113–22, 1978.

Peck, S. D., and Reiquam, C. W. Disseminated intravascular coagulation in cancer patients: supportive evidence. *Cancer* 31:1114–19, 1973.

FEVER

1) Malignancy

Fever associated with malignancy may be seen in patients with carcinoma (hypernephroma, liver, lung, gastrointestinal), melanoma, sarcoma (bone), lymphoma, and leukemia.

Treatment

Appropriate measures such as surgery, radiation therapy or chemotherapy should be instituted to control the underlying malignancy. Infection should be considered and treated promptly in febrile neutropenic patients with active leukemia or in febrile neutropenic patients who have just received chemotherapy.

2) Drug Fever

Drug fever may be induced by any of the commonly used drugs including antibiotics and chemotherapeutic agents. Chemotherapeutic agents which have been implicated include: bleomycin, imidazole carboxamide, doxorubicin, daunorobicin, L-asparaginase, 5-azacytidine, procarbazine, triethylenethiophosphoramide, mithramycin, methotrexate (including intrathecal) and BCG.

Treatment

Discontinue the offending agent. If symptoms persist or if the implicated drug must be continued, administer diphenhydramine (25–50 mg) and/or hydrocortisone (100 mg IV).

3) Transfusion Reaction

Transfusion reaction may occur following the administration of red blood cells, white blood cells or platelets and can be ascribed to immunity against antigens present on these agents.

Treatment

Slow or discontinue infusion. Administer diphenhydramine (25–50 mg) and/or hydrocortisone (100 mg IV). Meperidine (25–50 mg) may provide relief from shaking chills. Further laboratory work is required only if the reaction is unusually severe. Patients with antibodies against white blood cells or platelets may be given packed red blood cells with the buffer layer removed.

4) Infection

Fever from infection is seen in a wide variety of conditions: obstruction (biliary, renal, pulmonary), hypogammaglobulinemia (gram-positive organisms), reduced cell-mediated immunity, microorganisms (viruses, bacteria, fungi, parasites), and neutropenia due to myelosuppressive drugs or myelophthisis).

Treatment

Treatment of the specific underlying cause is indicated. Appropriate antibiotic, antifungal, or antiviral therapy should be instituted when indicated. Infection prophylaxis may be useful and may include protective isolation, gut sterilization with non-absorbable antibiotics (gentamicin, vancomycin, nystatin), vaccination with pneumococcal and influenza vaccines, trimethoprim-sulfamethoxazole, and granulocyte transfusion.

5) Collagen vascular disease

A variety of collagen vascular syndromes have been associated with malignancy and fever.

Treatment

Treatment consists of controlling the underlying malignancy. A trial dose of prednisone, 60–100 mg daily, may be effective.

References

Bodey, G. P.; Buckley, M.; Sathe, Y. S.; and Freireich, E. J. Quantitative relationships between circulating leukocytes and infection in patients with acute leukemia. *Ann. Intern. Med.* 64:328–40, 1966.

Boggs, D. R., and Frei, E. III. Clinical studies of fever and infection in cancer. *Cancer* 13:1240–53, 1960.

Browder, A. A.; Huff, J. W.; and Petersdorf, P. G. The significance of fever in neoplastic disease. *Ann. Intern. Med.* 55:932–42, 1961.

EORTC International Antimicrobial Therapy Project Group, The. Antibiotic regimens in the treatment of infection in febrile granulocytopenic patients with cancer. *J. Infect. Dis.* 137:14–29, 1978.

Ketchel, S. J., and Rodriguez, V. Acute infections in cancer patients. *Semin. Oncol.* 5:167–79, 1978.

Levine, A. S.; Schimpff, S. C.; Graw, R. G., Jr.; and Young, R. C.; Hematologic malignancies and other marrow failure states: progress in the management of complicateing infections. *Semin. Hematol.* 11:141–202, 1974.

Preisler, H. D., and Bjornsson, S. Protective environment units in the treatment of acute leukemia. *Semin. Oncol.* 2:369–77, 1975.

Schmipff, S. C.; Greene, W. H.; Young, W. M.; Fortner, C. L.; Jepsen, L.; Cusack, N.; Block, J. B.; and Wiernik, P. H. Infection prevention in acute nonlymphocytic leukemia. *Ann. Intern. Med.* 82:351–58, 1975.

MALIGNANT EFFUSIONS

1) Pleural Effusion

Pleural effusion can be seen in carcinoma (breast, lung), lymphoma, and mesothelioma. The characteristics of malignant effusion include low fluid glucose, positive cytology, exudative fluid (specific gravity greater than 1.015, fluid/serum protein ratio greater than 0.5, fluid LDH greater than 200 IV, and fluid/serum LDH greater than 0.6, chylous fluid, and an elevated carcinoembryonic antigen.

Treatment

Control of the underlying malignancy is essential. Complete drainage with thoracentesis should be attempted. Not more than 1000 cc of fluid should be removed at one time. Radiation therapy may be effective if administered as either an external beam or as radioisotopes. Nitrogen mustard or tetracycline instillation may be effective with frequent changes in position. Surgical approaches include pleurectomy and placement of a thoracostomy tube or pleural window.

2) Pericardial Effusion

Pericardial effusion may occur in lymphoma, carcinoma (lung, breast), mediastinal tumors or may be induced by radiation therapy. Cardiac tamponade may occur with as little as 250 ml of fluid or may involve 1000 ml or more. Clinical manifestations include dyspnea, orthopnea, tachycardia, reduced pulse pressure, increased venous pressure, paradoxical pulse, Kussmaul's sign, cardiomegaly, hepatic engorgement, and a positive hepatojugular reflex.

Treatment

Prompt measures should be undertaken. Pericardiocentesis under EKG monitor should be performed as an emergency procedure. External beam radiation therapy or placement of a pericardial window may then be considered. Refractory cases may require nitrogen mustard or tetracycline instillation. Prednisone (1 mg/kg) may be useful for radiation pericarditis. Efforts aimed at control of the underlying malignancy should be instituted.

3) Ascites

Ascites may occur in patients with carcinoma (ovarian) and lymphoma.

Treatment

Treatment should be directed at controlling the underlying malignancy. Paracentesis may be used diagnostically or therapeutically to relieve severe symptoms. In refractory cases, retroperitoneal radiation therapy or direct instillation of nitrogen mustard or tetracycline may be considered, but may be complicated by the risk of adhesions and intestinal obstruction.

NOTE: Methotrexate and other agents may sequester in effusions with subsequent prolonged release of the drug resulting in increased myelosuppression. Effusions due to infection, congestive heart failure or prior radiation therapy must be excluded.

References

Biran, S.; Brufman, G.; Klein, E.; et al. The management of pericardial effusion in cancer patients. *Chest* 71:182–86, 1977.

Chermow, B., and Sahn, S. A. Carcinomatous involvement of the pleura: an analysis of 96 patients. *Am. J. Med.* 63:695–702, 1977.

Davis, S.; Sharma, S. M.; Blumberg, E. D.; Kim, C. S. Intraparacardial tetracycline for tamponade secondary to malignant effusion. *N. Engl. J. Med.* 299:1113–14, 1978.

Izbicki, R., Weyhing, B. T. III; Baker, L.; Caoili, E. M.; and Vaitkevicius. V. K. Pleural effusion in cancer patients. *Cancer* 36:1511–18, 1975.

Leff, A.; Hopewell, P. C.; and Costello, J. Pleural effusion from malignancy. *Ann. Intern. Med.* 88:532–37, 1978.

Legha, S. S., and Muggia, F. M. Pleural mesothelioma: clinical features and therapeutic implications. *Ann. Intern. Med.* 87:613–21, 1977.

Light, R. W.; MacGregor, M. I.; Luchsinger, P. C.; and Ball, W. C. Jr. Pleural effusions: The diagnostic separation of transudates and exudates. *Ann. Intern. Med.* 77:507–13, 1972.

Rittgers, R. A.; Lowenstein, M. S.; Feinerman, A. E. et al: Carcinoembryonic antigen levels in benign and malignant pleural effusions. *Ann. Intern. Med.* 88:631–34, 1978.

Sarma, P.R., and Moore, M. R. Approach to the management of pleural effusion in malignancy. *South Med. J.* 71:133–40, 1978.

Theologies, A. Neoplastic cardiac tamponade. *Semin. Oncol.* 5:181–92, 1978.

Wallach, H. W. Intrapleural tetracycline for malignant pleural effusion. *Chest* 68:510–12, 1975.

MENTAL OBTUNDATION

1) Intracerebral Tumor

Mental obtundation may occur when an intracerebral lepto-meningeal tumor results in increased intracranial pressure or tentorial herniation.

Treatment

Maintain circulation and respiration while other measures are being instituted. Emergency treatment should include dexamethasone (10 mg IV stat and 4 mg every 6 hours), furosemide (40 mg IV every 6 hours), and mannitol (100 gm by IV infusion over 30 minutes). Definitive therapy may include craniotomy and/or radiaton therapy.

2) Intracranial Hemorrhage

Mental obtundation may occur from intracranial hemorrhage either as a result of spontaneous bleeding (intracerebral, subdural, spinal) or leukostasis (greater than 100,000 cells/cu. mm in peripheral blood).

Treatment

Platelet transfusion may be required. Blood pressure should be effectively reduced. Dexamethasone (10 mg IV stat and 4 mg every 6 hours) should be given. Analgesics and stool softeners may be helpful. Surgery may be required for spontaneous bleeding. Reduce the blast count with hydroxyurea, irradiate the brain in leukostasis, and avoid leukocyte transfusion.

3) Shock

Mental obtundation may occur in shock following sepsis or anaphylaxis.

Treatment

General measures for the treatment of shock should be instituted. Begin intravenous fluids to maintain urine output. Institute appropriate empiric antibiotic and steroid therapy for presumed sepsis. Vasopressor therapy may be required. Maintain proper oxygenation and acid-base balance. Use epinephrine (0.5 ml of 1:1000 soln. subcutaneously) and steroids (hydrocortisone 500 mg IV) for anaphylaxis.

4) Encephalopathy

Mental obtundation from encephalopathy may be due to radiation therapy, chemotherapy, viral infection, progressive multifocal leukoencephalopathy, cerebral demyelination, or metabolic and endocrine disorders.

Treatment

Treatment is directed at control of the underlying condition. Steroid therapy is of questionable benefit.

5) Infection

Mental obtundation may be due to systemic sepsis or central nervous system infection (meningitis, encephalitis).

Treatment

Initiate appropriate antibiotic therapy.

6) Hyperviscosity

Mental obtundation may occur with dysproteinemia.

Treatment

Initiate plasmapheresis in patients with viscosity greater than three. Chemotherapy for the underlying disorder may then be instituted.

7) Drug Induced

Drug induced CNS depression can result from a number of commonly used agents with CNS activity, including analgesics and antiemetics, as well as several chemotherapeutic agents (procarbazine, L-asparaginase).

Treatment

Withdraw the offending agent. Provide intravenous hydration, circulatory and ventilatory support. Consider the use of a narcotic antagonist (naloxone 0.4 mg IV) or hemodialysis if indicated.

NOTE: Proper care of the obtunded patient includes meticulous nursing care to prevent decubuti, corneal protection, indwelling catheters (if necessary), proper hydration and nutrition, and routine physical therapy. Insure airway patency and consider seizure precautions.

References

Chernik, N. L.; Armstrong, D.; and Posner, J. B. Central nervous system infections in patients with cancer. *Medicine* 52:563–81, 1973.

Goldsmith, M. A., and Carter, S. K. Glioblastoma multiforme. A review of therapy. *Cancer Treat. Rev.* 1:153–65, 1974.

McKee, J. C. Jr., and Collins, R. D. Intravascular leukocyte thrombi and aggregates as a cause of morbidity and mortality in leukemia. *Medicine* 53:463–78, 1974.

Posner, J. B. Neurological complications of systemic cancer. *Med. Clin. North Am.* 55:625–46, 1971.

Schnaper, N. Psychosocial aspects of management of the patient with cancer. *Med. Clin. North Am.* 61:1147–55, 1977.

PAIN

Pain in cancer patients may range from mild to severe and debilitating. Its presence may indicate the need for treatment of an underlying disorder. The reason for pain varies widely and may include such causes as obstruction, infection, inflammation, tissue destruction, and neurological compression. The control or relief of pain revolves around control of the underlying malignancy but may also include decompressive surgery, neurosurgical procedures, psychotherapy, biofeedback and hypnotic techniques, and analgesic drug therapy.

Several analgesic agents, combinations, and potentiators are listed below according to potency.

1) **Weak Analgesics**

acetylsalicylic acid:	300–600 mg q 4 h PO or PR
acetaminophen:	300–600 mg q 4 h PO or PR
propoxyphene:	65 mg q 4–6 h PO
pentazocine:	50 mg PO or 30 mg IM or IV q 4 h
codeine:	30–60 mg PO or 15–60 mg IM q 4 h

2) **Strong Analgesics**

meperidine:	50–100 mg PO or IM q 2–4 h
dihydromorphinone:	2–4 mg PO q 2–4 h
morphine sulfate:	5–15 mg IM or IV q 2–4 h
oxycodone and acetaminophen:	1–2 PO q 4–6 h
oxycodone and aspirin:	1–2 PO q 4–6 h

3) **Analgesic Potentiators**
   ethyl alcohol
   hydroxyzine
   phenothiazines
   tricyclic antidepressants

4) **Narcotic Analgesic Combinations** (formulations vary between institutions)

A) **Brompton's Cocktail** (example #1)

morphine sulfate	50–75 mg
cocaine hydrochloride	50 mg
chlorpromazine	75 mg
ethanol 95%	20 cc
syrup (flavored)	to make 100 cc

dose: 5–30 cc PO q 1–4 hours

B) **Brompton's Cocktail** (example #2)

morphine sulfate	50 mg
cocaine hydrochloride	50 mg
prochlorperazine	25 mg
distilled water	to make 100 cc

Dose: 5–30 cc PO q 1–4 hours

C) **Schlessinger's solution**

	per/drop	per/60 cc
scopolamine hydrobromide	0.125 mg	15 mg
morphine sulfate	2.0 mg	1.2 gm
ethylmorphine	4.0 mg	2.4 gm
distilled water	to make 1 drop	60 cc

dose: 2–5 drops PO q 2–4 hours in liquid

References

Gybels, J.; Adriaensen, H.; and Cosyns, P. Treatment of pain in patients with advanced cancer. *Eur. J. Cancer* 12:341–51, 1976.

Marks, R. M., and Sachar, E. J. Undertreatment of medical inpatients with narcotic analgesics. *Ann. Intern. Med.* 78:173–81, 1973.

Moertel, C. G.; Ahmann, D. L.; Taylor, W. F.; and Schwartow, N. A comparative evaluation of marketed analgesic drugs. *N. Engl. J. Med.* 286:813–15, 1972.

Mount, B. M.; Ajemian, I.; and Scott, J. F. Use of brompton mixture in treating the chronic pain of malignant disease. *Can. Med. Assoc. J.* 115:122–24, 1976.

Saunders, C. The treatment of intractable pain in terminal cancer. *Proc. R. Soc. Med.* 56:195–97, 1963.

TUMOR COMPRESSION

1) Spinal Cord Compression

Tumor compression may affect the spinal cord in the thoracic (70%), lumbosacral (20%) or cervical (10%) region. Underlying malignancies include lung, breast, lymphoma, myeloma, sarcoma, prostate, renal, gastrointestinal, and thyroid. This must be distinguished from viral or radiation-induced myelopathy.

Treatment

Treatment includes intensive supportive care and meticulous nursing care. Administer both dexamethasone (10 mg IV stat and 4 mg IV every 6 hours) and radiation therapy to the involved area. Rapid onset with a complete block necessitates decompressive laminectomy as an emergency procedure.

2) Nerve Root Compression

Nerve root compression may involve brachial plexus compression (breast, lung), Horner's syndrome (pancoast tumor), laryngeal nerve compression (lung, lymphoma), and peripheral nerve-pain syndrome. Distinguish nerve root compression from neuropathy due to carcinomatosis (lung, breast, ovary, lymphoma), drugs (vincristine), and from malignancy-induced myopathies (Eaton-Lambert Syndrome, polymyositis, and general wasting).

Treatment

Treatment is directed at the underlying malignancy with radiation therapy. Withhold vinca alkaloids. Initiate physical therapy to maintain muscle tone and prevent contractures.

3) Superior Vena Cava Syndrome

A superior vena cava syndrome may be seen in small cell carcinoma (40%), non-small cell bronchogenic carcinoma (40%), lymphoma (15%), and sarcoma. Superior vena cava compression may be a life-threatening complication of upper mediastinal malignancies.

Treatment

Administer dexamethasone (10 mg IV stat and 4 mg every 6 hours) and use oxygen as required for hypoxemia. Emergency radiation therapy may be required. Anticoagulants and fibrinolytic agents may be useful for associated thrombosis.

4) Visceral Obstruction

Respiratory distress due to lymphomas or bronchogenic carcinomas may result from compression of the larynx, hypopharynx, or trachea. Gastrointestinal obstruction may be due to primary malignancy or metastases at the level of the esophagus (melanoma or lymphoma of the breast, lung), stomach and small intestine (carcinoid of the pancreas, colon, ovary), or colon (ovary, cervix). Hepatobiliary obstruction may be either extrahepatic due to biliary tract or pancreatic carcinomas or lymphomas, or it may be intrahepatic due to carcinoma or drug-induced cholestasis. Chemotherapeutic agents associated with cholestasis include cyclophosphamide, L-asparaginase, 6-mercaptopurine, methotrexate, nitrosoureas, cytosine arabinoside, imidazole carboxamide, and mithramycin. Other drugs include the androgens, allopurinol, various antibiotics, and the phenothiazines. Genitourinary obstruction due to malignancy may occur at the ureteral level (lymphoma or sarcoma of the cervix, ovary, colon, prostate) or at the urethral level (prostate).

Treatment

Treatment consists of management of the underlying malignancy with surgical resection or bypass, radiotherapy, or chemotherapy. Respiratory airway patency should be maintained with tracheostomy if necessary. Esophageal dilation and intubation or gastroenterostomy may be necessary to maintain nutrition. Potential offending drugs should be withheld. Illeal-loop diversion, ureteral shunt, or nephrostomy may be necessary to relieve urinary obstruction. General measures include antibiotics for underlying infections, transfusions, and correction of electrolyte imbalances.

NOTE: When using drugs excreted primarily through the biliary tract, e.g., adriamycin and vinca alkaloids, an appropriate dose reduction should be made.

References

Bagley, F. H.; Walsh, J. W.; Cady, B.; et al. Carcinomatous versus radiation-induced brachial plexus neuropathy in breast cancer. *Cancer* 41:2154–57, 1978.

Bruckman, J. E., and Bloomer, W. D. Management of spinal cord compression. *Semin. Oncol.* 5:135–40, 1978.

Gilbert, R. W.; Kim, J. H.; and Posner, J. B. Epidural spinal cord compression from metastatic tumor: diagnosis and treatment. *Ann. Neuro.* 3:40–51, 1975.

Gomes, M. N., and Hufnagel, C. A. Superior vena cava obstruction. *Ann. Thorac. Surg.* 20:344–59, 1975.

Heal, J. M., and Schein, P. S. Management of gastrointestinal cancer. *Med. Clin. North Am.* 61:991–99, 1977

Jameson, R. M. Prolonged survival in paraplegia due to metastatic spinal tumors. *Lancet* 1:1209–11, 1974.

Perez, C. A.; Presant, C. A.; and Van Amburg, A. L. III. Management of superior vena cava syndrome. *Semin. Oncol.* 5:123–34, 1978.

Sise, J. G., and Chrichlow, R. W. Obstruction due to malignant tumors. *Semin. Oncol.* 5:213–24, 1978.

Welch, J. P. and Donaldson, G. A. Management of severe obstruction of the large bowel due to malignant disease. *Am. J. Surg.* 127:492, 1974.

METABOLIC DISORDERS

1) Cachexia

Cachexia may result from the systemic effects of malignancy, obstruction, malabsorption and hepatic dysfunction.

Treatment

Treatment consists of oral or nasogastric dietary supplementation, vitamins, and/or intravenous hyperalimentation, as well as treatment of the underlying malignancy.

2) Hypercalcemia

Hypercalcemia is seen with metastatic carcinoma (breast, lung, prostate) and multiple myeloma. Clinical manifestations include bone pain, dehydration, muscle weakness, apathy, obtundation, lengthened PR and QT intervals, polyuria, renal failure, nephrocalcinosis, nausea, constipation, pancreatitis, and metabolic alkalosis.

Treatment

Avoid immobilization, dehydration, and thiazide diuretics if possible to prevent hypercalcemia. For mild hypercalcemia (serum calcium 11–15 mg %) institute calcium restriction, increase fluid intake, and administer prednisone (1 mg/kg daily) and oral phosphate (1–3 gm daily).

In severe hypercalcemia (serum calcium greater than 15 mg %) give normal saline, furosemide (40–100 mg IV every 2–3 hours) and hydrocortisone (100 mg IV every 12 hours). Intravenous phosphate (1–1.5 gm over 6–8 hours) may be of some benefit. Mithramycin may be used in refractory hypercalcemia in intravenous doses of 25 mcg/kg every 1–2 days until serum calcium falls below 12 mg %.

3) Hyperuricemia

Hyperuricemia is seen in acute leukemia, lymphoma, and post-chemotherapy responsive malignancies. Clinical manifestations of hyperuricemia include gouty arthritis and urate nephropathy.

Treatment

Hyperuricemia is treated prophylactically with adequate hydration and allopurinol (300 mg PO daily). Significant hyperuricemia (uric acid greater than 8 mg/100 ml) requires intravenous fluids and alkalinization of the urine (sodium bicarbonate 16 gm daily or acetazolamide 0.5–2 gm daily) to prevent nephropathy. Uric acid nephropathy, once developed, may require hemodialysis until renal function improves.

4) Hyperkalemia

Hyperkalemia may be seen in patients with acute leukemia, lymphoma, and renal failure. The clinical manifestations of hyperkalemia include weakness, paralysis, bradycardia, hypotension, elevated T waves, depressed R waves, prolonged PR intervals, widened QRS and QT interval, and cardiac arrest.

Treatment

Mild hyperkalemia (K^+ 6–7 mEq/L) can be treated with cation exchange resins (removes approximately 1 mEq K^+/ gm). Severe hyperkalemia (K^+ greater than 7 mEq/L) can be treated with IV calcium gluconate, IV sodium bicarbonate, and/or 50 per cent glucose solution, and regular insulin.

5) Hypokalemia

Hypokalemia develops in patients with acute leukemia or in patients experiencing gastrointestinal loss of potassium (diarrhea, vomiting). The clinical manifestations of hypokalemia include weakness, paralysis, flat or inverted T wave, prominent U wave, and depressed ST segments, impaired renal concentrating ability, CNS symptoms and gastrointestinal symptoms.

Treatment

Mild hypokalemia is treated with potassium-rich foods (oranges, tomatoes, bananas) or potassium chloride 10% solution if necessary. Parenteral therapy may be required for severe hypokalemia. Potassium can be given at a rate of 10–40 mEq/hr IV in concentrations of 30-60 mEq/L. Not more than 100-200 mEq/day should be given.

6) Hypergammaglobulinemia

Hypergammaglobulinemia may be associated with the plasma cell dyscrasias (multiple myeloma, Waldenstrom's macroglobulinemia) or with various adenocarcinomas (colon, prostate, breast, lung).

Treatment

Symptoms related to hypergammagloblinemia and a viscosity greater than 3.0 should be treated by plasmapheresis. Chemotherapy for the underlying malignancy should be initiated concurrently.

7) Endocrine Disturbances

Endocrine abnormalities associated with cancer may develop as a result of a deficiency of hormone production (hypogonadism, hypothyroidism, adrenal insufficiency) or with the ectopic production of hormones. Ectopic hormone syndromes include the following conditions and their associated malignancies: Cushing's syndrome (small cell carcinoma, thymoma, islet cell carcinoma), syndrome of Inappropriate Antidiuretic Hormone (small cell carcinoma, thymoma, lymphoma, and gastrointestinal carcinomas, gynecomastia (bronchogenic carcinoma, hepatoma, adrenal carcinoma), hyperparathyroidism (hypernephroma, squamous cell lung cancer, pancreatic and ovarian adenocarcinoma), hyperthyroidism (choriocarcinoma, embryonal cell carcinoma), hypocalcemia (medullary carcinoma of the thyroid, breast carcinoma, small cell lung cancer), hypoglycemia (retroperitoneal sarcoma, islet cell carcinoma, hepatoma, adrenal cortical carcinoma, bronchogenic carcinoma), and hyperpigmentation (bronchogenic carcinoma).

Treatment

Treatment consists of management of the underlying malignancy. The syndrome of Inappropriate Antidiuretic Hormone results in hyponatremia that may require fluid restriction or hypertonic saline with concurrent diuresis. Hypocalcemia may require calcium dietary supplements or parenteral calcium gluconate. Hypoglycemia may require glucose administration. Diazoxide (150–450 mg IV) may be helpful in refractory insulinomas.

8) Cutaneous Changes

Cutaneous changes associated with malignancy may be a result of exposure to carcinogens, infiltration with tumor cells (breast and lung carcinomas, lymphoma, leukemia), infection, fat necrosis (pancreatic carcinoma), or associated endocrine or metabolic abnormalities (Addison's disease, melanoma, ancanthosis nigricans).

References

Besarab, A., and Caro, J. F. Mechanisms of hypercalcemia in malignancy. *Cancer* 41:2276–85, 1978.

Bower, B. F., and Gordan, G. S. Hormonal effects of nonendocrine tumors. *Ann. Rev. Med.* 16:83–118, 1965.

Deftos, L. J., and Neer, R. M. Medical management of the hypercalcemia of malignancy. *Ann. Rev. Med.* 25:323–31, 1974.

Dudrick, S. J.; Long, J. M.; Steiger, E.; and Rhoads, J. E. Intravenous hyperalimentation. *Med. Clin. North Am.* 54:577–89, 1970.

Greenberg, E.; Divertie, M. B.; and Woolner, L. B. A review of unusual systemic manifestations associated with carcinoma. *Am. J. Med.* 36:106–20, 1964.

Jones, S. E. Oncologic emergencies. *Arizona Med.,* 1976.

Kreisberg, R. A., and Pennington, L. F. Tumor hypoglycemia: a heterogeneous disorder. *Metabolism* 19:445–52, 1970.

Mazaferri, E. L.; O'Dorisio, T. M.; and LoBuglio, A. F. Treatment of hypercalcemia associated with malignancy. *Semin. Oncol.* 5:141–53, 1978.

Mir, M. A.; Brabin, B.; Tang, O. T., et al. Hypokalemia in acute myeloid leukemia. *Ann. Intern. Med.* 82:54–57, 1975.

Morrison, S. D. Partition of energy expenditure between host and tumor. *Cancer Res.* 31:98–107, 1971.

Samaan, N. A.; DeAssis, D. N.; Buzdar, A. U.; and Blemenschein, G. R. Pituitary-ovarian function in breast cancer patients on adjuvant chemotherapy. *Cancer* 41:2084–87, 1978.

Sherins, R. J.; Olweny, C. L.; and Ziegler, J. L. Gynecomastia and gonadal dysfunction in adolescent boys treated with combination chemotherapy for Hodgkin's disease. *N. Engl. J. Med.* 299:12–16, 1978.

Solomon, A. Homogenous (monoclonal) immunoglobulins in cancer. *Am. J. Med.* 63:169–76, 1977.

Theologides, A. A pathogenesis of cachexia in cancer. *Cancer* 29:484–88, 1972.

RESPIRATORY DISTRESS

1) Pulmonary Neoplasm

Pulmonary neoplasms may produce bronchial obstruction, massive parenchymal replacement, pulmonary effusion, and other complications contributing to respiratory distress.

Treatment

Treatment consists of control of the underlying malignancy with surgery, radiation therapy, and/or chemotherapy. Radiation therapy may relieve obstruction while thoracentesis, radiation therapy, and chemotherapy may be effective in the treatment of pleural effusions.

2) Pneumonia

Pneumonias of various etiologies must be considered as causes of respiratory distress. Infections produced by viruses, bacteria, fungi, and *Pneumocystis carinii* as well as pneumonias resulting from aspiration and radiation fibrosis may appear. Bleomycin, methotrexate, busulfan, and cyclophosphamide have been shown to be significant in the development of pneumonias related to the drugs' toxicities. Leukocyte transfusions may result in transient pulmonary infiltrates associated with respiratory distress.

Treatment

Underlying infection may be controlled by antibiotics and granulocyte transfusions in the refractory neutropenic patient. Aspiration pneumonias will respond to oxygenation, aminophylline for bronchospasms, antibiotics, and intravenous hydrocortisone if instituted early. If radiation fibrosis is suspected, prednisone (40–80 mg daily) may be administered as a therapeutic trial, although its value is questionable. Slow or stop leukocyte transfusion if respiratory distress occurs.

3) Congestive Heart Failure

Congestive heart failure may be seen as a consequence of overhydration, cardiovascular disease, and drug therapy. Doxorubicin, daunorubicin, cyclophosphamide, and radiation therapy have been implicated in the development of congestive heart failure.

Treatment

Congestive heart failure will respond to treatment with digoxin, 0.25 mg daily, furosemide, 40 to 80 mg daily, and fluid restriction. Pulmonary edema may require conventional emergency measures. Discontinue contributing agents.

4) Pulmonary Emboli

Pulmonary emboli must be considered in the differential diagnosis of respiratory distress resulting from chemotherapy.

Treatment

Generally accepted measures of treating pulmonary emboli, including continuous intravenous infusion of heparin followed by oral anticoagulation therapy, should be instituted immediately. Attempts to control the underlying malignancy will ultimately be the most beneficial.

NOTE: General measures to maintain airway patency, oxygenation, and ventilation should be taken. Other causes of respiratory distress, such as emphysema, pneumoconiosis, and pulmonary emboli, should be distinguished. Routine pulmonary physiotherapy is indicated in bedridden patients, individuals with COPD, and particularly in the neutropenic immunocompromised host. Postural drainage, proper humidification and hydration, deep breathing and coughing, percussion and vibration, and suctioning are essential, while mucolytic agents and bronchodilators may also be administered. Any patient exhibiting evidence of acute respiratory infection must be treated aggressively with appropriate antibiotics.

References

Blum, R.H.; Carter, S. K.; and Agre, K. A clinical review of bleomycin — a new antineoplactic agent. *Cancer* 31:903–04, 1973.

Bode, F. R.; Pare, A. P.; and Fraser, R. G. Pulmonary diseases in the compromised host. *Medicine* 53:255-93, 1974.

Farrell, J. T. Pulmonary metastases: a pathologic, clinical, roentgenologic study based on 78 cases seen at necropsy. *Radiology* 2:444–51, 1935.

Greenman, R. L.; Goodall, P. T.; and King, D. Lung biopsy in immunocompromised hosts. *Am. J. Med.* 59:488–96, 1975.

Rosenow, E. C. II. The spectrum of drug-induced pulmonary disease. *Ann. Intern. Med.* 77:977–91. 1972.

Sostman, H. D.; Matthay, R. A.; Putnam, C. E.; and Smith, G. J. W. Methotrexate-induced pneumonitis. *Medicine* 55:371–88, 1976.

Sostman, H. D.; Mathay, R. A.; and Putman, C. E. Cytotoxic drug-induced lung disease. *Am. J. Med.* 62:608–15, 1977.

Valdivieso, M.; Gil-Extremera, B.; Zornoza, J.; Rodriguez, V.; and Bodney, G. P. Gram-negative bacillary pneumonia in the compromised host. *Medicine* 56:241–54, 1977.

SHOCK (HYPOTENSION)

1) Sepsis

Sepsis must be considered in the differential diagnosis of shock.

Treatment

Management of sepsis and septic shock includes the administration of methyl-prednisolone, 30 mg/kg as an intravenous bolus followed by 100 mg intravenously every 4 hours. Appropriate antibiotic therapy for sepsis is essential.

2) Volume Depletion

Volume depletion may occur as a result of numerous processes and may precipitate shock. Gastrointestinal losses, including vomiting and diarrhea, and hemorrhage, third space accumulations (i.e. effusions), and fluid loss from conditions such as diabetes insipidus are possible etiologies of volume depletion leading to shock.

Treatment

Response is achieved with the administration of whole blood to actively bleeding patients while packed cells are indicated for slower bleeding if the hemoglobin is below 10 gm%. A fluid challenge with normal saline to maintain CVP above 15 cm of water may be considered. A daily oral dose of chlorpropamide or subcutaneous vasopressin will effectively manage diabetes insipidus. Paracentesis of ascitic fluid should only be considered for diagnostic purposes and relief of extreme discomfort.

3) Adrenal Insufficiency

Adrenal insufficiency is commonly encountered in patients treated for lung and breast cancer.

Treatment

Treatment may include administration of normal saline containing hydrocortisone and intramuscular cortisone acetate. Appropriate management of infection and hypokalemia is necessary.

4) Anaphylaxis

In addition to numerous other agents, L-asparaginase, bleomycin, and *cis*-platinum may precipitate anaphylaxis. Hypotension and shock have also been associated with 5-azacytidine, busulfan, and C. Parvum.

Treatment

Subcutaneous administration of 0.5 ml of a 1:1000 epinephrine solution will initiate emergency treatment. Saline infusion of 500 mg of intravenous aminophylline to maintain urine output and to alleviate bronchospasms, and 500 mg of hydrocortisone every 4 to 6 hours are necessary until a positive response is seen. Test doses of bleomycin and L-asparaginase are recommended before administration of therapeutic doses. Patients with a history of a prior allergic reaction should receive the Erwinia strain of L-asparaginase.

5) Cardiogenic Shock

Cardiogenic shock may be attributed to the use of doxorubicin, daunomycin, and high doses of cyclophosphamide.

Treatment

Initial management of cardiogenic shock is to withhold suspected drugs. Digoxin therapy, including loading and maintenance doses, must be initiated. Pulmonary edema necessitates aggressive treatment with oxygen, parenteral furosemide, rapid digitalization, rotating tourniquets, phlebotomy, and Swann-Ganz catheter monitoring where available.

6) Neurologic Shock

Possible etiologies of neurologic shock include spinal cord compression and peripheral neuropathy.

Treatment

Control of the underlying malignancy constitutes the most direct form of treatment. Decompressive laminectomy and/or radiation therapy must be considered a medical emergency.

NOTE: General measures must be instituted to restore plasma volume, maintain a CVP above 15 cm of water, and to correct the underlying condition. Restoration of blood pressure sufficient to maintain a urine output of at least 30 cc per minute (usually 90 to 100 mm Hg systolic blood pressure), must be pursued with vasopressors. Acidosis, hypoxia, and electrolyte disturbances must be concomitantly corrected.

References

Haskell, C. M.; Canellos, G. P.; Levanthal, B. G.; Carbone, P. P.; Block, J. B.; Serpick, A. A.; and Selwary, O. S. L-Asparaginase — therapeutic and toxic effects in patients with neoplastic disease. *N. Engl. J. Med.* 281:1028–34. 1969.

Schumer, W., and Nyhus, L. *Treatment of shock: principles and practice.* Philadelphia: Lea & Febiger, 1974.

VanHoff, D. D.; Rozencweig, M.; Layard, M.; Slavik, M.; and Muggia, F.M. Daunomycin-induced cardiotoxicity in children and adults: a review of 110 cases. *Am. J. Med.* 62:200–08, 1977.

VanHoff, D. D.; Slavik, M.; and Muggia, F. M. Letter: allergic reactions of *cis*-platinum. *Lancet* 1:90, 1976.

Whitecar, J. R., Jr.; Bodey, G. P.; Harris, J. E.; and Freireich, E. J. L-Asparaginase. *N. Engl. J. Med.* 282:732–34, 1970.

Yagoda, A.; Mukherji, B.; Young, C.; Etcubanas, E.; Lamonte, C.; Smith, J.; Tan, C. T. C.; and Krakoff, I. H. Bleomycin, an antitumor antibiotic. Clinical experience in 274 patients. *Ann. Intern. Med.* 77:861–70, 1972.

THROMBOEMBOLIC COMPLICATIONS

1) Carcinomatosis

This condition most commonly occurs in patients with pancreatic and other gastrointestinal malignancies.

Treatment

Treatment must be directed to the underlying malignancy wherever possible.

2) Disseminated Intravascular Coagulation (DIC)

The majority of patients with active malignancy exhibit subclinical DIC as evidenced by shortened fibrinogen survival. Clinical DIC is most frequently associated with acute leukemia and prostatic carcinoma or with sepsis accompanying the disorders.

Treatment

If the underlying etiology cannot be promptly corrected, continuous infusion of heparin should be considered. Replacement therapy with fresh-frozen plasma and platelets must also be considered. Prophylactic heparin (5 to 10 units/kg per hour by continuous infusion) is indicated for subclinical DIC associated with acute promyelocytic leukemia.

3) Hyperviscosity

Plasma cell dyscrasias and Waldenstrom's macroglobulinemia frequentlty result in clinically significant hyperviscosity.

Treatment

Plasmapheresis is indicated for symptoms of hyperviscosity and viscosity above 3, while treatment of the underlying condition is initiated.

4) Mixed Cryoglobulinemia

Common etiologies of mixed cryoglobulinemia include lymphomas, chronic lymphocytic leukemia, multiple myeloma, and macroglobulinemia.

Treatment

Successful treatment plans may include daily, oral doses of prednisone (40–60 mg) and/or a splenectomy.

5) Erythrocytosis

Erythrocytosis is present in cases of polycythemia rubra vera or it may occur secondarily to malignant or nonmalignant conditions, including renal, cerebellar or hepatocellular tumors, pheochromocytoma, uterine fibroma, adrenal adenoma, ovarian carcinoma, and rectal cancer.

Treatment

Phlebotomy is indicated in symptomatic patients and those with a hematocrit above 55%. Treatment approaches may include repeated phlebotomy or ^{32}Phosporus, oral alkylating agents.

6) Thrombocytosis

This disorder may be essential or associated with generalized malignancy including Hodgkin's disease and carcinomatosis or with myeloproliferative disorders such as CML, post splenectomy complications, sepsis, and iron deficiency.

Treatment

Management of any generalized malignancy is indicated while thrombocytopheresis, nitrogen mustard, busulfan, or chlorambucil constitute treatment of myeloproliferative disorders. Heparin, aspirin, and dipyridamole may be effective in preventing thrombosis.

NOTE: General measures for treating arterial occlusion include bedrest, heparin treatment (30,000–40,000 units IV daily by continuous infusion) antiplatelet or thrombolytic agents (dipyridamole, urokinase), and embolectomy when necessary. General measures for treating venous occlusion include bedrest, extremity elevation, heparin treatment. Prophylactic measures include antithrombotic stockings, low-dose heparin (5,000 units subcutaneously every 12 hours), early ambulation, and possibly antiplatelet agents.

References

Bloch, K. J., and Maki, D. G. Hyperviscosity syndromes associated with immunoglobulin abnormalities. *Semin. Hematol.* 10:133–134, 1973.

Mason, J. E.; DeVita V. T.; and Canellos, G. P. Thrombocytosis in chronic granulocytic leukemia: incidence and clinical significance. *Blood* 44:483–487, 1974.

Soloman, A., and Fahey, J. L. Plasmapheresis therapy in macroglobulinemia. *Ann. Intern. Med.* 58:789–800, 1963.

Waterbury, L. S., and Hampton, J. W. Hypercoagulability with malignancy. *Angiology* 18:197–203, 1967.

Wu, K. K. Platelet hyperaggregability and thrombosis in patients with thrombocythemia. *Ann. Intern. Med.* 88:7–11, 1978.

RENAL FAILURE

1) Renal Parenchymal Invasion

This process occurs most frequently in patients with acute leukemia and lymphoma.

Treatment

Systemic chemotherapy is essential in the treatment of renal parenchymal invasion while radiation therapy to the kidneys may also be considered.

2) Obstructive Uropathy

Ureteral obstruction may be present in cases of retroperitoneal tumors including lymphomas and sarcomas, and in cases of widespread carcinoma. Urethral obstruction is a frequently observed consequence of bladder and prostate carcinomas.

Treatment

It is necessary to treat the underlying malignancy, if feasible, with measures including surgical diversion, radiaton, and/or systemic chemotherapy.

3) Prerenal azotemia

Prerenal azotemia is a frequently observed consequence of sepsis, dehydration, and hypotension.

Treatment

Management considerations include a fluid challenge with normal saline to maintain an adequate CVP, appropriate antibiotics, and corticosteroids if indicated.

4) Drug-induced Renal Failure

Antibiotics, particularly gentamicin, tobramycin, cephalothin, and amphotericin B have been implicated in the development of renal failure. Nephrotoxicity is also attributable to numerous chemotherapeutic agents, notably *cis*-platinum, mithramycin, streptozotocin, mitomycin, and methotrexate.

Treatment

The initial treatment is to discontinue offending agents. Electrolytes and state of hydration must be monitored and managed with appropriate replacement therapy.

5) Hemolysis

Hemolysis may be seen as a reult of transfusions, drug administration, and disseminated intravascular coagulation (DIC).

Treatment

Potentially offending agents must be withheld and intravenous normal saline and mannitol are administered to maintain urine output at 50 - 100 cc per hour. DIC is appropriately managed by continuous heparin infusion.

6) Glomerulonephritis

Lipoid nephrosis may result from lymphoma, while immune-complex glomerulonephritis is often a consequence of colorectal, lung, and renal cell involvement. Amyloidosis is attributable to multiple myeloma or Waldenstrom's macroglobulinemia.

Treatment

Control of the underlying malignancy constitutes essential treatment while a trial of oral prednisone, 1 mg/kg per day, may also be beneficial.

7) Renal Vein Thrombosis

This complication is most frequently observed in patients with renal cell carcinoma and retroperitoneal metastases of carcinomas and lymphomas.

Treatment

Possible treatment plans include oral anticoagulants, antiplatelet agents, and thrombolytic therapy for refractory cases.

8) Myeloma Kidney

Myeloma kidney is distinguished by the presence of tubular casts of albumin, immunoglobulin, and light chains and may occur in patients with multiple myeloma, macroglobulinemia, and lymphoma.

Treatment

Hydration, particularly at night, and alkalinization with acetazolamide or sodium bicarbonate are beneficial, while hemodialysis and renal transplant constitute treatment of advanced disease.

9) Radiation nephritis

A latent period of 6 months or longer is observed before the development of radiation nephritis. This disorder is frequently complicated by hypertension.

Treatment

Intra-arterial epinephrine administered concomitantly with radiation therapy is a prophylactic measure that has been shown to decrease nephrotic damage. Hemodialysis and/or other supportive care is indicated in cases of radiation nephritis.

10) Metabolism

A variety of metabolic abnormalities associated with malignancy may result in renal dysfunction. These incude the following conditions and their associated malignancies: hypokalemia, hyperkalemia (leukemia, lymphoma), hypercalcemia (carcinoma of the breast and lung, multiple myeloma, leukemia, lymphoma), and hyperuricemia (leukemia, lymphoma), which may also occur following chemotherapy.

Treatment

Standard management methods for hypokalemia (KCl supplements), hyperkalemia (sodium polystyrene sulfanate or Kayexelate®, insulin, glucose), hypercalcemia (saline, diuretics, steroids), and hyperuricemia (urinary alkalinization, allopurinol) are indicated.

NOTE: The treatment of acute renal failure in cancer and in non-malignant disease is similar. Management of acidosis, electrolyte disturbances, volume overload, anemia, and complicating infections is essential. If necessary, hemodialysis and/or renal transplantation should be implemented.

References

Dahlgren, J. G.; Anderson, E. T.; and Hewitt, W. L. Gentamicin blood levels: A guide to nephrtoxicity. *Antimicrob. Agents Chemother.* 8:58–62, 1975.

DeFronzo, R. A.; Humphrey, R. L.; Wright, J. R.; and Cooke, C. R. Acute renal failure in multiple myeloma. *Medicine* 54:209–23, 1975.

Frei, E. III; Bentzel, C. J.; Rieselbach, R.; et al. Renal complications of neoplastic disease. *J. Chron. Dis.* 16:757–76, 1963.

Garnick, M. B., and Mayer, R. J. Acute renal failure associated with neoplastic diseases and its treatment. *Semin. Oncol.* 5:155–65, 1978.

Harrington, J. T., and Cohen, J. J. Current concepts: acute oliguria. *N. Engl. J. Med.* 292:89–91, 1975.

Hardaker, W. T., Jr.; Stone, R. A.; and McCoy, R. Platinum nephrotoxicity. *Cancer* 34:1030–32, 1974.

Rozencweig, M.; VanHoff, D. D.; Slavik, M.; and Muggia, F. M. *Cis*-diamminedichloroplatinum (II). *Ann. Intern. Med.* 86:803–12, 1977.

Slovin, S. F.; Graces, A.; Bennet, S. J.; and Pascal, R. R. Tumor-associated antibodies on glomerular basement membranes (GBM) of cancer patients. *Cancer Res.* 18:102, 1977.

Watts, R. W.; Walkins, P. J.; Matthias, J. Q.; et al. Allopurinol and acute uric acid nephropathy. *Brit. Med. J.* 1:205–208, 1966.

Appendix

Figure 1

NOMOGRAM

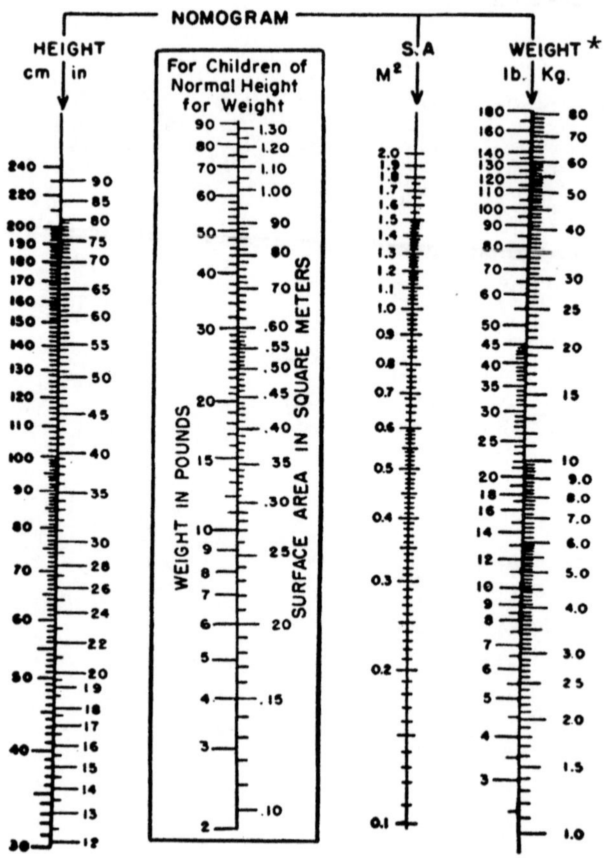

Nomogram for estimation of surface area. The surface area is indicated where a straight line, connecting the height and weight levels, intersects the surface area column. Average size, based on weight alone is indicated in the enclosed area. (Nomogram modified from data of E. Boyd by C.D. West.)

*Calculate on the basis of desirable body weight.

Note:

A straight edge is placed from the patient's height in the left column to his weight in the right column and this intersect on the body surface area column (S.A.) indicates his body surface area. For children of average build, the body surface area may be estimated from the weight alone by referring to the enclosed area in the left corner of the figure.

Formula used to convert mg/kg to mg/M^2:

Adults: $mg/kg \times 37 = mg/M^2$
Children: $mg/kg \times 25 = mg/M^2$

Source:

Textbook of Pediatrics, 10th ed., ed. V. C. Vaughan, III., M. D., R. J. McKay, M. D., and W. E. Nelson, M. D. (Philadelphia: W.B. Saunders Company, 1975).

Figure 2

Biochemical Sites of Action
Cancer Chemotherapeutic Agents

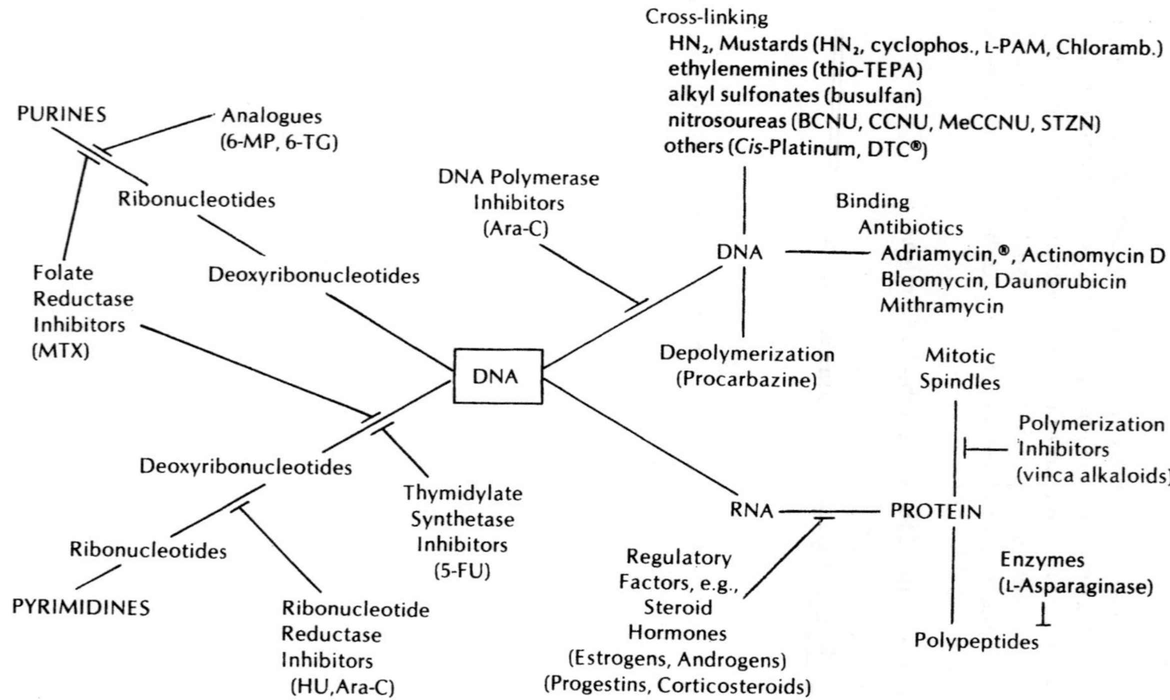

Table 1
Cancer Incidence by Site & Sex*

MALE	FEMALE
Skin 1%	Skin 1%
Oral 5%	Oral 2%
Lung 22%	Breast 26%
Colon & Rectum 14%	Lung 6%
Other Digestive 12%	Colon & Rectum 15%
Prostate 17%	Other Digestive 9%
Urinary 9%	Ovary 5%
Leukemia & Lymphomas 8%	Uterus 14%
All other 12%	Urinary 4%
	Leukemia & Lymphomas 7%
	All other 11%

Source: American Cancer Society 1977 Cancer Facts and Figures, 1976.

Excluding Non melanoma Skin cancer and carcinoma *in situ* of uterine cervix.

Table 2

Desirable Weight in Pounds and Kilograms (In Indoor Clothing)
Ages 25 and Over

Height (In Shoes)			Small Frame		Medium Frame		Large Frame	
ft	in	cm	lb	kg	lb	kg	lb	kg
Men								
5	2	157.5	112-120	50.8-54.4	118-129	53.5-58.5	126-141	57.2-64.0
5	3	160.0	115-123	52.2-55.8	121-133	54.9-60.3	129-144	58.5-65.3
5	4	162.6	118-126	53.5-57.2	124-136	56.2-61.7	132-148	59.9-67.1
5	5	165.1	121-129	54.9-58.5	127-139	57.6-63.0	135-152	61.2-68.9
5	6	167.6	124-133	56.2-60.3	130-143	59.0-64.9	138-156	62.6-70.8
5	7	170.2	128-137	58.1-62.1	134-147	60.8-66.7	142-161	64.4-73.0
5	8	172.7	132-141	59.9-64.0	138-152	62.6-68.9	147-166	66.7-75.3
5	9	175.3	136-145	61.7-65.8	142-156	64.4-70.8	151-170	68.5-77.1
5	10	177.8	140-150	63.5-68.0	146-160	66.2-72.6	155-174	70.3-78.9
5	11	180.3	144-154	65.3-69.9	150-165	68.0-74.8	159-179	72.1-81.2
6	0	182.9	148-158	67.1-71.7	154-170	69.9-77.1	164-184	74.4-83.5
6	1	185.4	152-162	68.9-73.5	158-175	71.7-79.4	168-189	76.2-85.7
6	2	188.0	156-167	70.8-75.7	162-180	73.5-81.6	173-194	78.5-88.0

6	3	190.5	160-171	72.6-77.6	167-185	75.7-83.5	178-199	80.7-90.3
6	4	193.0	164-175	74.4-79.4	172-190	78.1-86.2	182-204	82.7-92.5
				Women				
4	10	147.3	92- 98	41.7-44.5	96-107	43.5-48.5	104-119	47.2-54.0
4	11	149.9	94-101	42.6-54.8	98-110	44.5-49.9	106-122	48.1-55.3
5	0	152.4	96-104	43.5-47.2	101-113	45.8-51.3	109-125	49.4-56.7
5	1	154.9	99-107	44.9-48.5	104-116	47.2-52.6	112-128	50.8-58.1
5	2	157.5	102-110	46.3-49.9	107-119	48.5-54.0	115-131	52.2-59.4
5	3	160.0	105-113	47.6-51.3	110-122	49.9-55.3	118-134	53.5-60.8
5	4	162.6	108-116	49.0-52.6	113-126	51.3-57.2	121-138	54.9-62.6
5	5	165.1	111-119	50.3-54.0	116-130	49.0-59.0	125-142	49.4-64.4
5	6	167.6	114-123	51.7-55.3	120-135	54.4-61.2	129-146	58.5-66.2
5	7	170.2	118-127	53.5-57.6	124-139	56.2-63.0	133-150	60.3-68.0
5	8	172.7	122-131	55.3-59.4	128-143	58.1-64.9	137-154	62.1-69.9
5	9	175.3	126-135	57.2-61.2	132-147	59.9-66.7	141-158	64.0-71.7
5	10	177.8	130-140	59.0-63.5	136-151	61.7-68.5	145-163	65.8-73.9
5	11	180.3	134-144	60.8-65.3	140-155	63.5-70.3	149-168	67.6-76.2
6	0	182.9	138-148	62.6-67.1	144-159	65.3-72.1	153-173	69.4-78.5

SOURCE: Metropolitan Life Insurance Company, Weights of Insured Persons in the United States Associated with Lowest Mortality, November-December, 1959.

Table 3

Respective Surface Area To Weight Ratios (km) For Various Species

Species	Body Weight (kg)	Surface Area (sqm)	*km* Factor
Mouse	0.02	0.0066	3.0
Rat	0.15	0.025	5.9
Monkey	3.0	0.24	12
Dog	8.0	0.40	20
Human, child	20	0.80	25
Human, adult	60	1.60	37

Source:

E. J. Freireich *et al.*, Quantitative comparison of toxicity of anti-cancer agents in mouse, rat, dog, monkey and man. *Cancer Chemother. Rep.* 50(4):219–44, 1966.

Note:

To express a mg/kg dose in any given species as the equivalent mg/sqm dose, multiply the dose by the appropriate *km*. In the adult human, 100 mg/kg is equivalent to 100 mg/kg × 37 kg/sqm = 3700 mg/sqm.

Courtesy of National Cancer Institute. Chemotherapy, 1967.

Table 4

Equivalent Surface Area Dosage Conversion Factors

This table gives approximate factors for converting doses expressed in terms of mg/kg from one species to equivalent surface area doses expressed as mg/kg in the other species tabulated. The assumptions and constants presented in Freireich *et al.* (1966) are used.

		To			
	Mouse 20g	Rat 150g	Monkey 3.0kg	Dog 8kg	Man 60kg
From Mouse	1	1/2	1/4	1/5	1/12
Rat	2	1	1/2	1/4	1/7
Monkey	4	2	1	3/5	1/3
Dog	6	4	5/3	1	1/2
Man	12	7	3	2	1

Note:

Given a dose of 50 mg/kg in the mouse, what is the appropriate dose in the monkey, assuming equivalency on the basis of mg/M^2?

50 mg/kg × 1/4 = 13 mg/kg

Courtesy of National Cancer Institute. Chemotherapy, 1967.

Table 5

Surface area (m^2) as a funciton of height (inches) and weight (pounds)

Height (inches)	Weight (pounds)													
	10	15	20	25	30	35	40	45	50	55	60	65	70	75
20	0.27	0.33	0.38	0.43	0.47	0.51	0.55	0.58	0.62	0.65	0.68	0.70	0.73	0.76
22	0.28	0.34	0.40	0.45	0.49	0.53	0.57	0.61	0.64	0.67	0.70	0.73	0.76	0.79
24	0.29	0.36	0.41	0.47	0.51	0.55	0.59	0.63	0.66	0.70	0.73	0.76	0.79	0.82
26	0.30	0.37	0.43	0.48	0.53	0.57	0.61	0.65	0.69	0.72	0.76	0.79	0.82	0.85
28	0.31	0.38	0.44	0.50	0.55	0.59	0.63	0.67	0.71	0.75	0.78	0.81	0.84	0.87
30	0.32	0.39	0.46	0.51	0.56	0.61	0.65	0.69	0.73	0.77	0.80	0.84	0.87	0.90
32	0.33	0.40	0.47	0.53	0.58	0.62	0.67	0.71	0.75	0.79	0.82	0.86	0.89	0.92
34	0.34	0.41	0.48	0.54	0.59	0.64	0.69	0.73	0.77	0.81	0.85	0.88	0.92	0.95
36	0.34	0.42	0.49	0.55	0.61	0.66	0.70	0.75	0.79	0.83	0.87	0.90	0.94	0.97
38	0.35	0.43	0.50	0.57	0.62	0.67	0.72	0.76	0.81	0.85	0.89	0.92	0.96	0.99
	30	35	40	45	50	55	60	65	70	75	80	85	90	95
40	0.63	0.69	0.74	0.78	0.82	0.87	0.91	0.94	0.98	1.02	1.05	1.08	1.12	1.15
42	0.65	0.70	0.75	0.80	0.84	0.88	0.92	0.96	1.00	1.04	1.07	1.11	1.14	1.17
44	0.66	0.71	0.77	0.81	0.86	0.90	0.94	0.98	1.02	1.06	1.09	1.13	1.16	1.19
46	0.67	0.73	0.78	0.83	0.88	0.92	0.96	1.00	1.04	1.08	1.11	1.15	1.18	1.22
48	0.69	0.74	0.79	0.84	0.89	0.94	0.98	1.02	1.06	1.10	1.13	1.17	1.21	1.24
50	0.70	0.75	0.81	0.86	0.91	0.95	1.00	1.04	1.08	1.12	1.15	1.19	1.23	1.26
52	0.71	0.77	0.82	0.87	0.92	0.97	1.01	1.05	1.10	1.14	1.17	1.21	1.25	1.28
54	0.72	0.78	0.83	0.89	0.94	0.98	1.03	1.07	1.11	1.15	1.19	1.23	1.27	1.30
56	0.73	0.79	0.85	0.90	0.95	1.00	1.04	1.09	1.13	1.17	1.21	1.25	1.29	1.32
58	0.74	0.80	0.86	0.91	0.97	1.01	1.06	1.10	1.15	1.19	1.23	1.27	1.31	1.34
	50	60	70	80	90	100	110	120	130	140	150	160	170	180
60	0.98	1.08	1.16	1.25	1.32	1.40	1.47	1.54	1.60	1.66	1.72	1.78	1.84	1.89
62	0.99	1.09	1.18	1.26	1.34	1.42	1.49	1.56	1.62	1.69	1.75	1.81	1.86	1.92
64	1.01	1.11	1.20	1.28	1.36	1.44	1.51	1.58	1.65	1.71	1.77	1.83	1.89	1.94
66	1.02	1.12	1.21	1.30	1.38	1.46	1.53	1.60	1.67	1.73	1.79	1.85	1.91	1.97
68	1.03	1.13	1.23	1.31	1.40	1.47	1.55	1.62	1.69	1.75	1.82	1.88	1.94	2.00
70	1.04	1.15	1.24	1.33	1.41	1.49	1.57	1.64	1.71	1.78	1.84	1.90	1.96	2.02
72	1.06	1.16	1.26	1.35	1.43	1.51	1.59	1.66	1.73	1.80	1.86	1.92	1.98	2.04
	90	100	110	120	130	140	150	160	170	180	190	200	210	220
74	1.45	1.53	1.61	1.68	1.75	1.82	1.88	1.96	2.01	2.07	2.13	2.18	2.24	2.29
76	1.46	1.55	1.62	1.70	1.77	1.84	1.90	1.97	2.03	2.09	2.15	2.21	2.26	2.32
78	1.48	1.56	1.64	1.72	1.79	1.86	1.93	1.99	2.05	2.11	2.17	2.23	2.29	2.34
80	1.50	1.58	1.66	1.73	1.81	1.88	1.95	2.01	2.08	2.14	2.20	2.26	2.31	2.37
82	1.51	1.60	1.68	1.75	1.83	1.90	1.97	2.03	2.10	2.16	2.22	2.28	2.34	2.39
84	1.53	1.61	1.69	1.77	1.85	1.92	1.99	2.05	2.12	2.18	2.24	2.30	2.36	2.42
86	1.54	1.63	1.71	1.79	1.86	1.94	2.01	2.07	2.14	2.20	2.27	2.33	2.39	2.44

SOURCE: E. A. Gehan and S. L. George, Estimation of Human Body Surface Area from Height and Weight, *Cancer Chemother. Rep.* 54:225–35, 1970.

80	85	90	95	100	105	110	115	120	125
0.78	0.81	0.83	0.86	0.88	0.90	0.92	0.94	0.97	0.99
0.82	0.84	0.87	0.89	0.92	0.94	0.96	0.98	1.01	1.03
0.85	0.87	0.90	0.93	0.95	0.97	1.00	1.02	1.04	1.07
0.88	0.90	0.93	0.96	0.98	1.01	1.03	1.06	1.08	1.10
0.90	0.93	0.96	0.99	1.01	1.04	1.06	1.09	1.11	1.14
0.93	0.96	0.99	1.02	1.04	1.07	1.10	1.12	1.15	1.17
0.96	0.99	1.02	1.04	1.07	1.10	1.13	1.15	1.18	1.20
0.98	1.01	1.04	1.07	1.10	1.13	1.16	1.18	1.21	1.23
1.00	1.04	1.07	1.10	1.13	1.16	1.18	1.21	1.24	1.26
1.03	1.06	1.09	1.12	1.15	1.18	1.21	1.24	1.27	1.29

100	105	110	115	120	125	130	135	140	145
1.18	1.21	1.24	1.27	1.29	1.32	1.35	1.38	1.40	1.43
1.20	1.23	1.26	1.29	1.32	1.35	1.38	1.40	1.43	1.46
1.23	1.26	1.29	1.32	1.35	1.38	1.40	1.43	1.46	1.49
1.25	1.28	1.31	1.34	1.37	1.40	1.43	1.46	1.49	1.51
1.27	1.31	1.34	1.37	1.40	1.43	1.46	1.49	1.51	1.54
1.30	1.33	1.36	1.39	1.42	1.45	1.48	1.51	1.54	1.57
1.32	1.35	1.38	1.41	1.45	1.48	1.51	1.54	1.57	1.59
1.34	1.37	1.41	1.44	1.47	1.50	1.53	1.56	1.59	1.62
1.36	1.39	1.43	1.46	1.49	1.52	1.55	1.59	1.62	1.64
1.38	1.41	1.45	1.48	1.51	1.55	1.58	1.61	1.64	1.67

190	200	210	220	230	240	250	260	270	280
1.95	2.00	2.05	2.10	2.15	2.19	2.24	2.29	2.33	2.38
1.97	2.03	2.08	2.13	2.18	2.23	2.27	2.32	2.36	2.41
2.00	2.05	2.11	2.16	2.21	2.26	2.30	2.35	2.40	2.44
2.03	2.08	2.13	2.18	2.24	2.28	2.33	2.38	2.43	2.47
2.05	2.11	2.16	2.21	2.26	2.31	2.36	2.41	2.46	2.50
2.08	2.13	2.19	2.24	2.29	2.34	2.39	2.44	2.49	2.54
2.10	2.16	2.21	2.27	2.32	2.37	2.42	2.47	2.52	2.57

230	240	250	260	270	280	290	300	310	320
2.35	2.40	2.45	2.50	2.55	2.60	2.64	2.69	2.74	2.78
2.37	2.43	2.48	2.53	2.58	2.63	2.67	2.72	2.77	2.81
2.40	2.45	2.50	2.55	2.61	2.65	2.70	2.75	2.80	2.84
2.42	2.48	2.53	2.58	2.63	2.68	2.73	2.78	2.83	2.87
2.45	2.50	2.56	2.61	2.66	2.71	2.76	2.81	2.86	2.90
2.48	2.53	2.58	2.64	2.69	2.74	2.79	2.84	2.89	2.93
2.50	2.56	2.61	2.66	2.71	2.77	2.82	2.87	2.91	2.96

Table 6

Surface area (m²) as a function of height (cm) and weight (kg)

Height (cm)	Weight (kg)													
	4	6	8	10	12	14	16	18	20	22	24	26	28	30
50	0.25	0.31	0.36	0.40	0.44	0.48	0.51	0.54	0.57	0.60	0.63	0.66	0.68	0.71
55	0.26	0.32	0.37	0.42	0.46	0.50	0.53	0.57	0.60	0.63	0.66	0.68	0.71	0.74
60	0.27	0.33	0.39	0.43	0.48	0.52	0.55	0.59	0.62	0.65	0.68	0.71	0.74	0.76
65	0.28	0.34	0.40	0.45	0.49	0.53	0.57	0.61	0.64	0.67	0.70	0.73	0.76	0.79
70	0.29	0.36	0.41	0.46	0.51	0.55	0.59	0.63	0.66	0.69	0.73	0.76	0.79	0.81
75	0.30	0.37	0.42	0.48	0.52	0.57	0.61	0.64	0.68	0.71	0.75	0.78	0.81	0.84
80	0.31	0.38	0.44	0.49	0.54	0.58	0.62	0.66	0.70	0.73	0.77	0.80	0.83	0.86
85	0.31	0.39	0.45	0.50	0.55	0.60	0.64	0.68	0.72	0.75	0.79	0.82	0.85	0.88
90	0.32	0.40	0.46	0.51	0.56	0.61	0.65	0.70	0.73	0.77	0.81	0.84	0.87	0.91
95	0.33	0.40	0.47	0.53	0.58	0.63	0.67	0.71	0.75	0.79	0.83	0.86	0.89	0.93
	12	14	16	18	20	22	24	26	28	30	32	34	36	38
100	0.59	0.64	0.68	0.73	0.77	0.81	0.84	0.88	0.91	0.95	0.98	1.01	1.04	1.07
105	0.60	0.65	0.70	0.74	0.78	0.82	0.86	0.90	0.93	0.97	1.00	1.03	1.06	1.09
110	0.61	0.67	0.71	0.76	0.80	0.84	0.88	0.92	0.95	0.99	1.02	1.05	1.08	1.11
115	0.63	0.68	0.73	0.77	0.81	0.86	0.89	0.93	0.97	1.00	1.04	1.07	1.10	1.13
120	0.64	0.69	0.74	0.79	0.83	0.87	0.91	0.95	0.99	1.02	1.06	1.09	1.12	1.15
125	0.65	0.70	0.75	0.80	0.84	0.89	0.93	0.97	1.00	1.04	1.07	1.11	1.14	1.17
130	0.66	0.71	0.77	0.81	0.86	0.90	0.94	0.98	1.02	1.06	1.09	1.13	1.16	1.19
135	0.67	0.73	0.78	0.83	0.87	0.92	0.96	1.00	1.04	1.07	1.11	1.15	1.18	1.21
140	0.68	0.74	0.79	0.84	0.89	0.93	0.97	1.01	1.05	1.09	1.13	1.16	1.20	1.23
145	0.69	0.75	0.80	0.85	0.90	0.94	0.99	1.03	1.07	1.11	1.14	1.18	1.22	1.25
	30	34	38	42	46	50	54	58	62	66	70	74	78	82
150	1.12	1.20	1.27	1.34	1.40	1.46	1.52	1.58	1.63	1.69	1.74	1.79	1.84	1.88
155	1.14	1.21	1.29	1.35	1.42	1.48	1.54	1.60	1.65	1.71	1.76	1.81	1.86	1.91
160	1.15	1.23	1.30	1.37	1.44	1.50	1.56	1.62	1.68	1.73	1.78	1.84	1.89	1.94
165	1.17	1.25	1.32	1.39	1.46	1.52	1.58	1.64	1.70	1.75	1.81	1.86	1.91	1.96
170	1.18	1.26	1.34	1.41	1.48	1.54	1.60	1.66	1.72	1.78	1.83	1.88	1.94	1.99
175	1.20	1.28	1.35	1.43	1.49	1.56	1.62	1.68	1.74	1.80	1.85	1.91	1.96	2.01
180	1.21	1.29	1.37	1.44	1.51	1.58	1.64	1.70	1.76	1.82	1.88	1.93	1.98	2.04
	40	44	48	52	56	60	64	68	72	76	80	84	88	92
185	1.42	1.49	1.56	1.63	1.69	1.75	1.81	1.87	1.93	1.98	2.03	2.08	2.13	2.18
190	1.44	1.51	1.58	1.65	1.71	1.77	1.83	1.89	1.95	2.00	2.06	2.11	2.16	2.21
195	1.45	1.53	1.60	1.67	1.73	1.79	1.85	1.91	1.97	2.02	2.08	2.13	2.18	2.23
200	1.47	1.54	1.62	1.68	1.75	1.81	1.87	1.93	1.99	2.05	2.10	2.15	2.21	2.26
205	1.49	1.56	1.63	1.70	1.77	1.83	1.89	1.95	2.01	2.07	2.12	2.18	2.23	2.28
210	1.50	1.58	1.65	1.72	1.79	1.85	1.91	1.97	2.03	2.09	2.14	2.20	2.25	2.30
215	1.52	1.59	1.67	1.74	1.80	1.87	1.93	1.99	2.05	2.11	2.17	2.22	2.27	2.33
220	1.53	1.61	1.68	1.75	1.82	1.89	1.95	2.01	2.07	2.13	2.19	2.24	2.30	2.35

SOURCE: E. A. Gehan and S. L. George, Estimation of Human Body Surface Area from Height and Weight, *Cancer Chemother. Rep.* 54:225–35, 1970.

32	34	36	38	40	44	48	52	56	60
0.73	0.75	0.78	0.80	0.82	0.86	0.90	0.94	0.97	1.01
0.76	0.78	0.81	0.83	0.85	0.90	0.94	0.98	1.01	1.05
0.79	0.81	0.84	0.86	0.88	0.93	0.97	1.01	1.05	1.09
0.82	0.84	0.87	0.89	0.91	0.96	1.00	1.05	1.09	1.13
0.84	0.87	0.89	0.92	0.94	0.99	1.04	1.08	1.12	1.16
0.87	0.89	0.92	0.95	0.97	1.02	1.07	1.11	1.16	1.20
0.89	0.92	0.95	0.97	1.00	1.05	1.10	1.14	1.19	1.23
0.91	0.94	0.97	1.00	1.02	1.08	1.13	1.17	1.22	1.26
0.94	0.97	0.99	1.02	1.05	1.10	1.15	1.20	1.25	1.29
0.96	0.99	1.02	1.05	1.07	1.13	1.18	1.23	1.28	1.32

40	42	44	48	52	56	60	64	68	72
1.10	1.13	1.15	1.21	1.26	1.30	1.35	1.40	1.44	1.48
1.12	1.15	1.18	1.23	1.28	1.33	1.38	1.43	1.47	1.52
1.14	1.17	1.20	1.25	1.31	1.36	1.41	1.45	1.50	1.55
1.16	1.19	1.22	1.28	1.33	1.38	1.43	1.48	1.53	1.58
1.19	1.22	1.24	1.30	1.36	1.41	1.46	1.51	1.56	1.60
1.21	1.24	1.27	1.32	1.38	1.43	1.49	1.54	1.58	1.63
1.23	1.26	1.29	1.35	1.40	1.46	1.51	1.56	1.61	1.66
1.25	1.28	1.31	1.37	1.43	1.48	1.53	1.59	1.64	1.69
1.26	1.30	1.33	1.39	1.45	1.50	1.56	1.61	1.66	1.71
1.28	1.32	1.35	1.41	1.47	1.53	1.58	1.64	1.69	1.74

86	90	94	98	102	106	110	114	118	122
1.93	1.98	2.02	2.07	2.11	2.15	2.19	2.23	2.27	2.31
1.96	2.00	2.05	2.09	2.14	2.18	2.22	2.26	2.30	2.34
1.98	2.03	2.08	2.12	2.17	2.21	2.25	2.29	2.34	2.38
2.01	2.06	2.10	2.15	2.19	2.24	2.28	2.32	2.37	2.41
2.04	2.08	2.13	2.18	2.22	2.27	2.31	2.35	2.40	2.44
2.06	2.11	2.16	2.20	2.25	2.30	2.34	2.38	2.43	2.47
2.09	2.13	2.18	2.23	2.28	2.32	2.37	2.41	2.45	2.50

96	100	104	108	112	116	120	124	128	132
2.23	2.28	2.33	2.37	2.42	2.46	2.50	2.55	2.59	2.63
2.26	2.31	2.35	2.40	2.44	2.49	2.53	2.58	2.62	2.66
2.28	2.33	2.38	2.43	2.47	2.52	2.56	2.60	2.65	2.69
2.31	2.36	2.40	2.45	2.50	2.54	2.59	2.63	2.68	2.72
2.33	2.28	2.43	2.48	2.52	2.57	2.62	2.66	2.70	2.75
2.36	2.41	2.45	2.50	2.55	2.60	2.64	2.69	2.73	2.77
2.38	2.43	2.48	2.53	2.58	2.62	2.67	2.71	2.76	2.80
2.40	2.45	2.50	2.55	2.60	2.65	2.69	2.74	2.79	2.83

GPSR Compliance

The European Union's (EU) General Product Safety Regulation (GPSR) is a set of rules that requires consumer products to be safe and our obligations to ensure this.

If you have any concerns about our products, you can contact us on ProductSafety@springernature.com

In case Publisher is established outside the EU, the EU authorized representative is:

Springer Nature Customer Service Center GmbH
Europaplatz 3
69115 Heidelberg, Germany

Batch number: 10620163

Printed by Printforce, the Netherlands